Diabetic

MW00513932

2020

*The Perfect Step-by-Step Guide for the
Preparation of Healthy, Detoxifying and
Fat-Free Meals, Ideal for People with
Diabetes Problems + Daily Food Plan*

Isabella Williams

© **Copyright 2020 – Isabella Williams - All rights reserved.**

The content contained within this book may not be reproduced, duplicated, or transmitted without direct written permission from the author or the publisher.

Under no circumstances will any blame or legal responsibility be held against the publisher, or author, for any damages, reparation, or monetary loss due to the information contained within this book, either directly or indirectly.

Legal Notice:

This book is copyright protected. It is only for personal use. You cannot amend, distribute, sell, use, quote or paraphrase any part, or the content within this book, without the consent of the author or publisher.

Disclaimer Notice:

Please note the information contained within this document is for educational and entertainment purposes only. All effort has been executed to present accurate, up to date, reliable, complete information. No warranties of any kind are declared or implied. Readers acknowledge that the author is not engaging in the rendering of legal, financial, medical or professional advice. The content within this book has been derived from various sources. Please consult a licensed professional before attempting any techniques outlined in this book.

By reading this document, the reader agrees that under no circumstances is the author responsible for any losses, direct or indirect, that are incurred as a result of the use of the information contained within this document, including, but not limited to, errors, omissions, or inaccuracies.

Table of contents

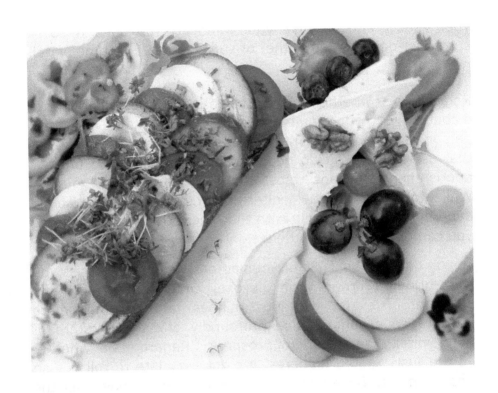

Introduction

Individuals with diabetes have almost twofold the danger of coronary illness and are at more risk of creating psychological wellness issues, for example, grief. Be that as it may, most instances of type 2 diabetes are preventable, and some can even be tacked. Finding a way to forestall or control diabetes doesn't mean living in hardship; it implies eating a scrumptious, adjusted eating routine that will likewise help your vitality and improve your mindset. You don't need to surrender desserts altogether or surrender to a lifetime of dull nourishment.

Regardless of whether you're attempting to forestall or control diabetes, your wholesome needs are equivalent to every other person, so no extraordinary nourishments are essential. Be that as it may, you do need to focus on a portion of your nourishment decisions—most eminently the starches you eat. While following a the Mediterranean or other heart-sound eating regimens can help with this, the most significant thing you can do is to lose a little weight.

Losing only 5% to 10% of your all-out weight can assist you with bringing down your glucose, circulatory strain, and cholesterol levels. Getting thinner and eating more advantageous can likewise profoundly affect your state of mind, vitality, and feeling of prosperity. Regardless of whether you've just created diabetes, it's not very late to roll out an improvement. By eating more advantageous, being all the more physically dynamic, and getting thinner, you can diminish your manifestations or even turn around diabetes. Most importantly, you have more authority over your wellbeing than you might suspect.

And that is why this cookbook is crafted and is focused on improving the lives of individuals living with diabetes and the individuals who bolster them. You are our anxiety, our center, and our central goal. To help you in dealing with your diabetes, or that of a friend or family member, we offer this assortment of plans, contributed by individuals from the council, the staff of Evergreen Clinic, and other minding individuals in the Evergreen people group. We comprehend that overseeing diabetes, regardless of whether it is your very own or that of somebody in your family, requires additional consideration and tirelessness.

With the correct frame of mind, backing, and toolbox, it tends to be controlled for a long, healthy, and fulfilling life. Diabetes requires executives, not really hardship. This cookbook is another device to assist you in withholding your diabetes under tight restraints. Simultaneously, notwithstanding, we trust that it rouses you to discover the joy in cooking for yourself as well as other people and to discover different wellsprings of inventive and scrumptious plans that are additionally predictable with a solid eating routine.

Cooking isn't just engaging, yet it enables you to find a workable pace individual with the fixings that will eventually support your body and your life. Solid weight control plans are for those with diabetes, yet the entire family. We are not merely offering diet plans that are carb-cognizant and bravo. These are additionally a portion of our preferred dishes, and we trust that you appreciate them as much as we do. Suppers are an open door for shared understanding. We unequivocally urge you to cook with and for your loved ones. Another vast apparatus is to design your menu on a week by week premise. Knowing early what you will prepare and eat enables you to stock your home with high fixings. Shopping supper by-dinner requires significantly more exertion and empowers motivation purchasing that can bring about poor choices. Utilize these plans and others that you find for designing your dinners and assuming responsibility for your eating routine. Embracing a conscious and principled way to deal with dinner arranging and nourishment buys will deliver considerable profits in wellbeing and diabetes control. We trust that you appreciate these plans as much as we do. Attempt them, exchange them, and make your stock of delectable and sound suppers.

Glycemic list and burden

A few people who have diabetes utilize the glycemic record to choose nourishments, particularly sugars. This well-prepared starch-containing nourishments are dependent on their impact on blood glucose levels. Chat with your dietitian about whether this technique may work for you.

Starches (carbs) are the essential nourishment that raises glucose. Glycemic record and glycemic load are logical terms used to quantify the effect of starch on glucose.

Nourishments with low glycemic load (a record) raise glucose unobtrusively and, in this manner, are better decisions for individuals with diabetes. The fundamental factors that decide a nourishment's (or meal's) glycemic load are the measure of fiber, fat, and protein it contains.

The distinction between glycemic record and glycemic load is that the glycemic list is a standardized estimation, and glycemic load represents an actual bit size. For instance, the glycemic file of a bowl of peas is 68 (per 100 grams), yet its glycemic load is only 16 (bring down the better). If you just alluded to the glycemic record, you'd think peas were an awful decision, however, as a general rule, and you wouldn't eat 100 grams of peas. With an average bit size, peas have a stable glycemic load just as being a great wellspring of protein.

Simple Diabetes Diet Myths

A diabetic eating regimen doesn't need to be muddled, and you don't need to surrender all your preferred nourishments. The initial step to settling on more intelligent decisions is to isolate the legends from the realities about eating to forestall or control diabetes.

Essential Diabetes Nourishment Myths You Shouldn't Accept

With all the data out there on how you ought to or shouldn't eat, it's anything but difficult to become involved with bogus data. Here are a few legends to disregard, beginning at this point:

You can never have your preferred nourishments again. False — regardless of whether it's a sugary cupcake or white bread. "Albeit nobody should make these nourishments a customary piece of their dinner plan, there are no food sources that are completely beyond reach with diabetes," Palinski-Swim says.

Sugar is awful. Eat close to 10 percent of your all-out calories from included sugars, Palinski-Swim prescribes. This is the same as the rules for everybody, which means you can at present appreciate a couple of chomps of pastry on the off chance that you'd like.

You shouldn't eat Fruits. The positive news about berries, apples, and melons (notwithstanding various sorts of fruits) is that they contain wellbeing advancing nutrients, cell reinforcements, and fiber calls attention to Palinski-Swim. A natural product can be a piece of your diabetes diet.

It would be best if you made yourself a different meal. Diabetes isn't a sentence to eat exhausting, tasteless nourishments. You can eat similar nourishment as your family, and even include uncommon food sources to a great extent, as indicated by the Joslin Diabetes Center. Below are a few more fantasies and realities of some meals to eat and avoid as a diabetes patient:

Fantasy: You should maintain a strategic distance from sugar no matter what.
For real: You can make the most of your preferred treats as long as you plan appropriately and limit concealed sugars. Treat doesn't need to be beyond reach, as long as it's a piece of a sound dinner plan.

Fantasy: You need to chop route down on carbs.
For real: The kind of starches you eat just as serving size is vital. Concentrate on entire grain carbs rather than bland carbs since they're high in fiber and processed gradually, keeping glucose levels all the more even.

Fantasy: You'll need exceptional diabetic dinners.
For Real: The standards of proper dieting are the equivalent—regardless of whether you have diabetes. Costly diabetic nourishments, for the most part, offer no exceptional advantage.

Fantasy: A high-protein diet is ideal.
For real: Studies have indicated that eating an excess of protein, particularly creature protein, may cause insulin obstruction, a critical factor in diabetes. A solid eating regimen incorporates protein, starches, and fats. However, our bodies need all of the three to work appropriately. The key is a reasonable eating regimen.
Similarly, as with any smart dieting program, a diabetic eating routine is more about your general dietary example instead of fixating on explicit nourishments. Plan to eat increasingly regular, natural nourishment and less bundled and comfort nourishments.

Regularly You are expected to Eat more

- Sound fats from nuts, olive oil, fish oils, flax seeds, or avocados
- Products of the soil—in a perfect world crisp, the more beautiful, the better; entire organic product as opposed to juices
- High-fiber oats and bread produced using whole grains
- Fish and shellfish, natural chicken or turkey
- Top-notch protein, for example, eggs, beans, low-fat dairy, and unsweetened yogurt

You are expected to Eat less

- Trans fats from in part hydrogenated or southern style nourishments
- Bundled and quick nourishments, particularly those high in sugar, heated products, desserts, chips, sweets
- White bread, sugary grains, refined pasta or rice
- Handled meat and red meat
- Low-fat items that have supplanted fat with included sugar, for example, sans fat yogurt
- Pick high-fiber, slow-discharge carbs

Starches significantly affect your glucose levels—more so than fats and proteins—so you should be shrewd about what kinds of carbs you eat. Cutoff refined carbohydrates like white bread, pasta, and rice, just as pop, sweets, bundled suppers, and nibble nourishments. Concentrate on high-fiber complex starches—otherwise called moderate discharge carbs. They are processed all the more gradually in this manner, keeping your body from creating an excess of insulin.

Be keen about desserts

Eating a diabetic eating regimen doesn't mean dispensing with sugar out and out; however, like the majority of us, odds are you expend more sugar than is sound. On the off chance that you have diabetes, you can, at present, appreciate a little serving of your preferred sweet once in a while. The key is balance.

Decrease your yearnings for desserts by gradually lessen the sugar in your eating routine a little at once to give your taste buds time to alter.
Hold the bread (or rice or pasta) on the off chance that you need dessert. Eating desserts at dinner includes additional starches, so cut back on the other carb-substantial nourishments at a similar supper.

Add some solid fat to your pastry. Fat hinders the stomach related procedure, which means glucose levels don't spike as fast. That doesn't mean you should go after the doughnuts, however. Think solid fats, for example, nutty spread, ricotta cheddar, yogurt, or nuts.
Eat desserts with a supper, instead of as an independent tidbit. When eaten without anyone else, sweets cause your glucose to spike. However, on the off chance that you eat them alongside other solid nourishments as a significant aspect of your feast, your glucose won't ascend as quickly.

At the point when you eat dessert, appreciate each chomp. How frequently have you carelessly eaten your way through a sack of treats or a colossal bit of cake? Will you truly state that you delighted in each nibble? Make the most of your guilty pleasure by eating gradually and focusing on the flavors and surfaces. You'll appreciate it progressively, in addition to you're more reluctant to indulge.

Simple Ways To Eliminate Body Blood Sugar

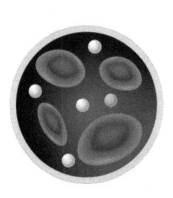

NORMAL LEVEL

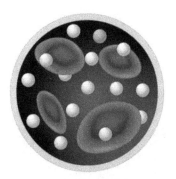

HYPERGLYCEMIA
(high blood sugar)

Decrease sodas, pop, and squeeze: For every 12 oz. serving of a sugar-improved refreshment you drink a day, your hazard for diabetes increments by around 15 percent. Take a stab at shining water with a bit of lemon or lime. Cut down on flavors and sugars you add to tea and espresso.

Try not to supplant saturated fat with sugar: A significant number of us supplant saturated fat, for example, entire milk dairy with refined carbs, believing we're settling on a more favorable decision. Low-fat doesn't mean sound when the fat has been supplanted by included sugar.

Improve nourishments yourself: Purchase unsweetened frosted tea, plain yogurt, or unflavored cereal, for instance, and include sugar (or organic product) yourself. You'll likely add far less sugar than the producer.

Check names and select low sugar items and utilize crisp or solidified fixings rather than canned merchandise. Be particularly mindful of the sugar substance of grains and sugary beverages.

Keep away from prepared or bundled nourishments like canned soups, solidified suppers, or low-fat dinners that frequently contain shrouded sugar. Plan more suppers at home.

Decrease the measure of sugar in Diet plans by ¼ to ⅓: You can support sweetness with mint, cinnamon, nutmeg, or vanilla concentrate rather than sugar.

Find reliable approaches to fulfill your sweet tooth: Rather than a dessert, mix up solidified bananas for a smooth, solidified treat. Or then again appreciate a little piece of dull chocolate, as opposed to a milk chocolate bar.

Start with half of the pastry you ordinarily eat and supplant the other half with fruits.

Be cautious about liquor: It's anything but difficult to think little of the calories and carbs in mixed beverages, including lager and wine. What's more, mixed drinks blended in with pop and squeeze can be stacked with sugar. Pick without calorie blenders, drink just with nourishment, and screen your blood glucose as liquor can meddle with diabetes drug and insulin.

Spot concealed sugar: Being savvy about desserts is just a piece of the fight. Sugar is likewise covered up in many bundled nourishments, inexpensive food suppers, and supermarket staples, for example, bread, grains, canned products, pasta sauce, margarine, moment pureed potatoes, solidified meals, low-fat dinners, and ketchup. The initial step is to spot concealed sugar on nourishment marks, which can take some sleuthing:

Makers give the aggregate sum of sugar on their marks; however, they don't need to separate between included sugar and sugar that is generally in the nourishment.

Included sugars are recorded in the fixings yet aren't in every case effectively unmistakable accordingly. While sugar, nectar, or molasses are sufficiently simple to spot, included sugar could likewise be recorded as corn sugar, high-fructose corn syrup, vanished stick juice, agave nectar, stick precious stones, alter sugar, or any fructose, dextrose, lactose, maltose, or syrup.

While you'd anticipate that sugary nourishments should have sugar recorded close to the highest priority on their rundown of fixings, producers frequently utilize various sorts of included sugars, which at that point seem dispersed down the review. Be that as it may, all these little portions of various sugars can signify a ton of added sugar and void calories!

Precautions should be taken with Fatty Foods
While Fatty foods are not bad, there are some that are dangerous to health, especially to a diabetic patient, and others have massive medical advantages, so it's essential to pick fats carefully.

Healthy fats: The most beneficial fats are unsaturated fats, which originate from fish and plant sources, for example, olive oil, nuts, and avocados. Omega-3 unsaturated fats battle aggravation and bolster the mind and heart wellbeing. Excellent sources incorporate salmon, fish, and flaxseeds.

Unhealthy fats: The most harming fats are fake trans fats, which make vegetable oils more averse to ruin. Stay away from monetarily heated products, bundled nibble nourishments, singed nourishment, and anything with "somewhat hydrogenated" oil in the fixings, regardless of whether it professes to be trans without fat.

Pure fats: Found for the most part in tropical oils, red meat, and dairy, there's no compelling reason to kill immersed fat from your eating regimen—but instead, appreciate with some restraint. The American Diabetes Affiliation prescribes expending close to 10% of your day by day calories from saturated fat.

Approaches to reduce unhealthy fats and retain Healthy fats:

Rather than chips or wafers, nibble on nuts or seeds or add them to your morning grain. Nut spreads are likewise fulfilling. Rather than fricasseeing, decide to sear, prepare, or pan sear. Maintain a strategic distance from immersed fat from prepared meats, bundled dinners, and takeout nourishment. Rather than merely red meat, shift your eating regimen with skinless chicken, eggs, fish, and veggie lover wellsprings of protein.

Utilize extra-virgin olive oil t dress servings of mixed greens, cooked vegetables, or pasta dishes.
Serving of mixed greens dressings is regularly high in calories, and trans fat, so make your own with olive oil, flaxseed oil, or sesame oil. Add avocados to sandwiches and plates of mixed greens or make guacamole.

Alongside being stacked with solid fats, they make for a filling and fulfilling feast. Be careful with dairy products.

Eat routinely and keep your diet plan Handy

It's urging to realize that you need to lose 7% of your body weight to slice your danger of diabetes down the middle. What's more, you don't need to check calories or starve yourself to do it fanatically. Two of the most accommodating procedures include following a standard eating calendar and recording what you eat.

Eat at consistently set occasions

Your body is better ready to manage glucose levels—and your weight—when you keep up a standard supper plan. Focus on moderate and reliable segment sizes for every supper.

Start your day away from work with a decent breakfast. It will give vitality just as relentless glucose levels.
Eat standard little suppers—up to 6 every day. Eating routinely will assist you in holding your parts in line.
Keep calorie admission the equivalent. To direct glucose levels, attempt to eat generally a similar sum each day, instead of indulging one day or at one supper, and afterward holding back the following.

Keep a Dieting Plan
An ongoing report found that individuals who kept a nourishment journal lost twice as a lot of weight as the individuals who didn't. Why? A setup account encourages you to distinguish issue regions, for example, your evening nibble or your morning latte—where you're getting a more significant number of calories than you understood. It likewise builds your familiarity with what,

why, and the amount you're eating, which causes you to cut back on thoughtless nibbling.

Get increasingly dynamic
Exercise can assist you in dealing with your weight and may improve your insulin affectability. A simple method to begin practicing is to stroll for 30 minutes every day (or for three 10-minute sessions if that is simpler). You can likewise take a stab at swimming, biking, or some other moderate-power action that makes them burn some serious calories and breathing harder.

No nourishment is untouchable when you have diabetes. The key is to watch divides, balance what you eat, and have about a similar number of starches in every feast. These four hints can assist you with the beginning, alongside formula thoughts for breakfast, lunch, and supper.

Test your glucose levels to figure out how various nourishments influence them.
Adhere to a specific number of sugar grams per feast. Typically this is around 45-75 grams three times each day.

Offset carbs with fiber and protein in every supper. This is simple if you utilize the plate technique. Make half of your plate vegetables, a fourth of your plate a carb like darker rice, dark beans, or entire wheat pasta, and the other quarter of your plate a substantial protein like chicken bosom, fish, lean meat, or tofu. Include a few products of the soil low-fat or sans fat milk or yogurt, contingent upon your carb focus for that dinner.

Eat brilliant fats, for example, those in nuts, avocado, fish, olives, and different plants. Maintain a strategic distance from immersed fats from meat, margarine, cheddar, and other dairy nourishments. Note: Coconut, albeit a plant, has saturated fat.

If any of the plans beneath has fewer carbs than what your PCP or human services group has prescribed per dinner, balance the feast with more carbs. This could incorporate nonfat yogurt or milk, products of the soil, or a little bit of entire grain bread.

Factors that Influence your Glucose Level As a Diabetes Patient

Keeping your glucose levels inside the range suggested by your PCP can be testing. That is on the grounds that numerous things make your glucose levels change, at times out of the blue. Following are a few factors that can influence your glucose levels.

Exercise

Physical action is another significant piece of your diabetes executive plan. At the point when you work out, your muscles use sugar (glucose) for vitality. Standard physical movement likewise enables your body to utilize insulin all the more productively.

These variables cooperate to bring down your glucose level. The more strenuous your exercise, the more drawn out the impact keeps going. Be that as it may, even light exercises —, for example, housework, planting, or being on your feet for broadened periods — can improve your glucose.

Steps to Follow:
Converse with your primary care physician about an activity plan. Get some information about what kind of activity is fitting for you. When all is said in done, most grown-ups should practice at any rate 30 minutes per day on most days of the week. On the off chance that you've been idle for quite a while, your PCP might need to check your general wellbeing before prompting you. The person in question can prescribe the correct parity of oxygen-consuming and muscle-fortifying activity.

Keep an activity plan: Converse with your primary care physician about the best time of day for you to practice, so your exercise routine is composed of your feast and medicine plans.

Know your numbers. Converse with your primary care physician about what glucose levels are fitting for you before you start work out.

Check your glucose level: Check your glucose level previously, during, and after exercise, mainly if you take insulin or prescriptions that lower glucose. Exercise can bring down your glucose levels even after a day, particularly if the action is different from you, or in case you're practicing at an increasingly escalated level. Know about admonition indications of low glucose, for example, feeling unsteady, powerless, worn out, eager, bleary-eyed, bad-tempered, on edge, or befuddled.

If you use insulin and your glucose level is below 100 milligrams for every deciliter (mg/dL), or 5.6 millimoles per liter (mmol/L), have a little nibble before you start practicing to forestall a low glucose level.

Remain hydrated: Drink a lot of water or different liquids while practicing in light of the fact that drying out can influence glucose levels.

Be readied: Continuously have a little tidbit or glucose tablets with you during exercise on the off chance that your glucose level drops excessively low. Wear a therapeutic distinguishing proof armlet when you're working out.

Change your diabetes treatment plan varying. On the off chance that you take insulin, you may need to lessen your insulin portion before working out or stand by for a short time after exercise to infuse insulin. Your primary care physician can advise you on suitable changes in your drug. You may likewise need to alter treatment if you've expanded your activity schedule.

Nourishment

Smart dieting is a foundation of stable living — with or without diabetes. However, in the event that you have diabetes, you have to know how nourishments influence your glucose levels. It's the kind of nourishment you eat, as well as the amount you eat and the blends of nourishment types you eat.

Steps to Follow:
Find out about starch tallying and divide sizes: The key to a well planned life as a patient is figuring out how to count starches. Carbohydrates are the nourishments that regularly have the most significant effect on your glucose levels. What's more, for individuals taking supper time insulin, it's vital to know the measure of starches in your nourishment, so you get the best possible insulin portion.

Identify what part size is fitting for each kind of nourishment: Disentangle your dinner arranging by recording divides for the nourishments you eat frequently. Use estimating cups or a scale to guarantee legitimate part size and a precise starch check.

Make each dinner well-adjusted: However, much as could reasonably be expected, plan for each dinner to have a decent blend of starches, foods grown from the ground, proteins, and fats. It's particularly critical to focus on the sorts of sugars you pick. A few sugars, for example, natural products, vegetables, and entire grains are preferable for you over are others. These nourishments are low in starches and contain fiber that helps keep your glucose levels progressively steady. Converse with your primary care physician, attendant, or dietitian about the best nourishment decisions and the proper parity of nourishment types.

Facilitate your dinners and meds: Too little nourishment concerning your diabetes meds — particularly insulin — may bring about perilously low glucose (hypoglycemia). An excess of food may cause your glucose level to climb excessively high (hyperglycemia). Converse with your diabetes social insurance group about how to best arrange supper and medicine plans.

Stay away from sugar-improved drinks: Sugar-improved refreshments — incorporating those improved with high fructose corn syrup or sucrose — will, in general, be high in calories and offer little in the method for sustenance. What's more, since they cause glucose to rise rapidly, it's ideal to stay away from these sorts of beverages in the event that you have diabetes.

The particular case is on the off chance that you are encountering a low glucose level. Sugar-improved refreshments, for example, pop, squeeze, and sports drinks can be utilized as a compelling treatment for rapidly raising excessively low glucose.

Medicine

Insulin and different diabetes drugs are intended to bring down your glucose levels when diet and exercise alone aren't adequate for overseeing diabetes. Be that as it may, the adequacy of these meds relies upon the planning and size of the portion. Prescriptions you take for conditions other than diabetes additionally can influence your glucose levels.

Steps to Follow:
Store insulin appropriately. Insulin that is inappropriately put away or past its lapse date may not be viable. Insulin is particularly touchy to limits in temperature.

Report issues to your primary care physician: In the event that your diabetes prescriptions cause your glucose level to drop excessively low or if it's reliably too high, the dose or timing may be balanced.

Be wary of new meds: In case you're thinking about an over-the-counter prescription or your primary care physician recommends another medication to treat another condition —, for example, hypertension or elevated cholesterol — ask your PCP or drug specialist if the medicine may influence your glucose levels. Fluid drugs might be improved with sugar to cover their taste. Some of the time a substitute medicine might be suggested. Continuously check with your primary care physician before taking any new over-the-counter prescription, so you know how it might affect your glucose level.

Disease

At the point when you're wiped out, your body produces pressure related hormones that help your body battle the sickness, yet they likewise can raise your glucose level. Changes in your craving and typical movement also may entangle diabetes on the board.

Steps to Follow:

Plan ahead: Work with your medicinal services group to make a day off arrangement. Remember guidelines for what drugs to take, how frequently to quantify your glucose and pee ketone levels, how to change your prescription measurements, and when to call your primary care physician.

Keep on taking your diabetes drug: In any case, in case you can't eat on account of sickness or regurgitating, contact your PCP. In these circumstances, you may need to modify your insulin portion or briefly quit taking your drug in light of the danger of hypoglycemia.

Adhere to your diabetes supper plan: On the off chance that you can, eating as regular will assist you with controlling your glucose levels. Keep a stock of nourishments that are simple on your stomach, for example, gelatin, saltines, soups, and fruit purée. Drink heaps of water or different liquids that don't include calories, for example, tea, to ensure you remain hydrated. In case you're taking insulin, you may need to taste sugar-improved refreshments, for example, juice or a games drink, to prevent your glucose level from dropping excessively low.

Alcohol

The liver regularly discharges put away sugar to balance falling glucose levels. In any case, if your liver is caught up with utilizing liquor, your glucose level may not get the lift it needs from your liver. Alcohol can bring about low glucose not long after you drink it and for upwards of 24 hours more.

Steps to Follow:

Get your PCP's alright to drink liquor. Liquor can disturb diabetes confusions, for example, nerve harm and eye illness. However, on the off chance that your diabetes is leveled out and your primary care physician concurs, an incidental mixed beverage is fine. Moderate liquor utilization is characterized as close to one beverage daily for ladies of all ages and men more than 65 years of age and two beverages every day for men under 65. One drink raises to a 12-ounce lager, 5 ounces of wine, or 1.5 ounces of refined spirits.

Try not to drink mixed refreshments on an unfilled stomach: If you take insulin or different diabetes drugs, make sure to eat before you drink or drink with dinner to forestall low glucose.

Pick your beverages cautiously: Light brew and dry wines have fewer calories and sugars than do other mixed drinks. In the event that you lean toward blended beverages, without sugar blenders —,, for example, diet pop, diet tonic, club pop, or seltzer — won't raise your glucose.

Count your calories: Make sure to incorporate the calories from any liquor you drink in your day by day carbohydrate level. Ask your primary care physician or dietitian how to join calories and starches from mixed beverages into your eating regimen plan.

Check your glucose level before bed: Since liquor can bring down glucose levels long after you've had your last beverage, check your glucose level before you rest. If your glucose isn't somewhere in the range of 100 and 140 mg/dL (5.6 and 7.8 mmol/L), have a bite before bed to counter a drop in your glucose level.

Feminine cycle and menopause

Changes in hormone levels the prior week and during the female period can bring about noteworthy vacillations in glucose levels. What's more, in a couple of years prior and during menopause, hormone changes may bring about flighty varieties in glucose levels that entangle diabetes the board.

Steps to Follow:
Search for designs. Monitor your glucose readings from month to month. You might have the option to foresee variances identified with your menstrual cycle.

Alter your diabetes treatment plan varying. Your primary care physician may prescribe changes in your dinner plan, activity level, or diabetes meds to compensate for glucose variety.

Check glucose all the more frequently. In case you're likely moving toward menopause or encountering menopause, converse with your primary care physician about whether you have to screen your glucose level all the more regularly. Indications of menopause can, in some cases, be mistaken for side effects of low glucose, so at whatever point conceivable, check your glucose before getting a presumed low affirm the low glucose level.

Ladies with diabetes can utilize most types of anti-conception medication without an issue. Be that as it may, oral contraceptives may bring glucose to step up in certain ladies.

Stress

In case you're focused on the hormones your body creates because of delayed pressure may cause an ascent in your glucose level. Also, it might be more enthusiastically to intently follow your standard diabetes the executives routine in case you're under a ton of additional weight.

Steps to Follow:
Log your feeling of anxiety on a size of 1 to 10 each time you log your glucose level. An example may occur before a long rise.

Take control: When you realize how stress influences your glucose level, retaliate. Learn unwinding strategies, organize your undertakings, and set points of confinement. At whatever point conceivable, evade regular stressors. Exercise can frequently help assuage pressure and lower your glucose level.

Find support: Adopt new techniques for adapting to pressure. You may locate that working with a therapist or clinical social laborer can assist you with distinguishing stressors, take care of distressing issues or change new adapting aptitudes.

The more you think about components that impact your glucose level, the more you can envision variances — and plan appropriately. In case you're experiencing difficulty keeping your glucose level in your objective range, approach your diabetes social insurance group for help.

Fruits And Vegetables

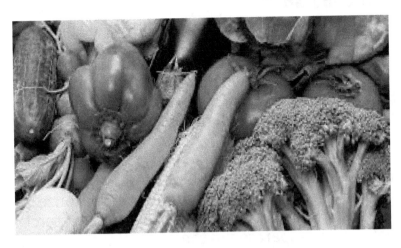

High-supplement, low glycemic load (GL) nourishments are the ideal food sources for people with diabetes. Furthermore, these nourishments likewise help to prevent and maintain diabetes in any case.

Vegetables

Supplement thick green vegetables – verdant greens, cruciferous vegetables, and other green vegetables – are the most significant nourishments to concentrate on for diabetes counteraction and inversion. Higher green vegetable utilization is related to a lower danger of creating type 2 diabetes, and among people with diabetes, higher green vegetable admission is related to lower HbA1c levels.

An ongoing meta-investigation found that more prominent verdant green admission was related to a 14% reduction in the danger of type 2 diabetes.

One examination announced that every day by day serving of verdant greens creates a 9% decline in chance.

Non-Green Vegetables

Non-green, non-boring vegetables like mushrooms, onions, garlic, eggplant, peppers, and so forth are fundamental segments of a diabetes counteraction (or inversion) diet. These nourishments have practically nonexistent impacts on blood glucose and have vast amounts of fiber and phytochemicals.

Beans

Lentils, beans, and different vegetables are the perfect starch source. They're low in glycemic load because of their moderate protein and copious fiber and safe starch, sugars that are not separated in the small digestive tract. This diminishes the measure of calories from the beans; besides, safe starch experiences aging by microscopic organisms in the colon, shaping items that secure against colon malignant growth. In like manner, bean and vegetable utilization are related to decreased danger of both diabetes and colon malignancy.

Nuts and Seeds

Wealthy in fiber and cancer prevention agents, natural products are a thick supplement decision for fulfilling sweet yearnings.

Eating three servings of crisp natural products every day is related to an 18% lessening in danger of diabetes. For the individuals who now have diabetes, I prescribe adhering to low sugar natural products like berries, kiwi, oranges, and melon to limit glycemic impacts.
Low in glycemic burden, nuts and seeds advance weight reduction, and have calming impacts that may forestall the improvement of insulin opposition.

The Medical caretakers' Wellbeing Concentrate found a 27% diminished danger of diabetes in attendants who ate at least five servings of nuts for every week. Among medical attendants who previously had diabetes, this equivalent amount decreased the danger of coronary illness by 47%.

Chia seeds

Chia is a kind of seed that gives fiber, protein, and omega-3 unsaturated fats. Chia is a superfood because it cuts down the glycemic heap of any supper, builds hunger fulfillment (satiety), and settles blood sugar. Adding chia to your morning meal will help keep you full more. The essential kind of fiber in chia is dissolvable fiber. Solvent filaments go to a gel when blended in with water. This makes chia seeds magnificent to use in preparing and cooking when a thickener is required. Chia blended in with almond milk, cocoa, and a low-glycemic list sugar like agave or stevia makes a great sound pudding!

Wild salmon

Salmon is a sort of diabetes superfood because salmon is an incredible wellspring of calming omega-3 unsaturated fats. There are contrasts in the unsaturated fats in the wild versus cultivated salmon. This is a result of what the fish eat. Wild salmon eat littler fish and live in colder waters, which makes them build up a higher proportion of calming omega-3s to immersed fats in their meat. Cultivated fish are up to multiple times higher in diligent natural toxins, anti-microbials, and different contaminants. These harmful synthetic compounds are star incendiary and have been related to an expanded danger of malignant growth and coronary illness.

White balsamic vinegar

The superfood vinegar is best expended as vinaigrette dressing on your plate of mixed greens, yet it has beneficial impacts regardless of how you appreciate it. Vinegar eases back gastric discharging, which has a few gainful implications for individuals with type 2 diabetes. This reduces back the glucose discharge into the circulatory system, taking into consideration a little, consistent insulin reaction rather than an enormous insulin flood. Vinegar likewise expands satiety, so on the off chance that you appreciate serving of mixed greens with vinaigrette as your first course, you are more averse to gorge during the principle course.

Cinnamon

Cinnamon brings down the blood glucose level in individuals with type 2 diabetes, and it has been very much investigated and saw as valuable at dosages of around 1 teaspoon/day.
Cinnamon brings down both fasting and postprandial (after suppers) glucose levels.

It is anything but difficult to add to any dietary example.
- Cinnamon can be sprinkled on cereal.
- It likewise is delicious added to espresso!
- Its high polyphenol content likewise has included advantage in forestalling wellbeing entanglements.

Lentils

Lentils are a superfood on the grounds that they contain significant nutrients, have incredible protein, and have loads of fiber. Lentils are creamy in iron, different minerals, and B nutrients, for example, folate. Lentils have an incredible parity of protein and complex sugar (high in fiber) and are incredibly flexible to cook with.

The green and dark-colored ones remain firm when cooked and are delectable in a serving of mixed greens. The orange ones get delicate when cooked, making them appropriate in Indian soups, curries, and dal.

Prepared carbs (white bread, pasta, chips, saltines)

Trans fats (anything with the word hydrogenated on the mark, for example, margarine "spreads," some mayonnaise "spreads" some plate of mixed greens dressings, bundled sauces, pastry shop merchandise.

The ideal approach to maintain a strategic distance from these nourishments is to search around the edges of the supermarket and limit the quantity of handled, bundled nourishments in the center. Staying with "genuine" nourishment in its entire, insignificantly controlled structure is an ideal approach to eat well for diabetes. Individuals with type 2 diabetes who eat a sound eating regimen design like the ones talked about here decrease the danger of inconveniences that come from high glucose, as cardiovascular malady and weight.

Recipes

Breakfast Recipes

Breakfast Wrap

Ingredients:

1 Egg, 3 Egg Whites

Low-carb Flour Tortilla

¼ Cleaved tomato

Onions

¼ Avocado

1/8 Fat Chaddar

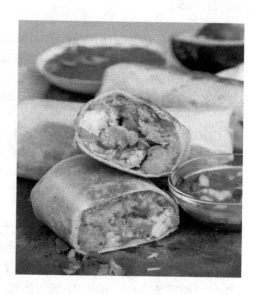

Descriptions:

Scramble 1 egg and 2 egg whites (or 1/4 cup egg substitute) in a little non-stick skillet covered with cooking shower. On a microwave-safe plate, spread the cooked eggs down the focal point of a multigrain or low-carb flour tortilla. Top with wanted trimmings, for example, 1/4 cup cleaved tomato, slashed green onion, 1/4 avocado, or 1/8 cup pasted fat cheddar. Microwave on high for around 20 seconds to relax the tortilla and warm the filling. Wrap up and appreciate it.

Evaluation: Starches 30g - Protein 18g - Fiber 6g

Coconut Quinoa Formula

Ingredients

1 cup quinoa

1 Can (13 to 15 oz) coconut milk (normal or light)

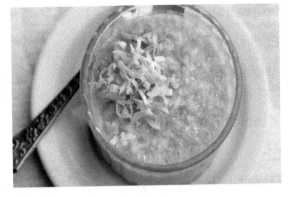

1 cup of water

1 teaspoon cinnamon

1 teaspoon vanilla concentrate

1 Tablespoon unadulterated maple syrup

Discretionary garnishes: bananas, berries, coconut drops, cut nuts, and so forth

Descriptions

Join all fixings (aside from discretionary garnishes) in a medium sized pot. Heat the blend to the point of boiling. Then reduce the heat to a minimal point, and then leave the quinoa to stew for at least 20-25 minutes; turn the mixture to blend periodically until delicate and thicken. Serve quickly or store in a refrigerator and warmth up later or serve cold.

Nutritional Evaluation:

Sugars 45g

Protein 10g

Fat 10g

Fiber 7g

English Wheat Biscuit

Ingredients:

English Wheat Biscuit

1 tablespoon of normal Spread

1 tablespoon of Jam

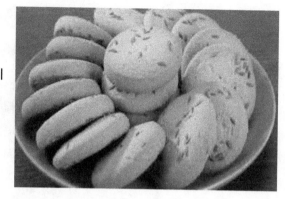

Descriptions:

Toast an entire wheat English biscuit and spread 1 tablespoon common style nutty spread on one half and 1 tablespoon less-sugar jam on the other half. Appreciate with an entire bit of fruits, like, an orange or banana.

Nutritional Evaluation:

Sugars 47g

Protein 10g

Fiber 7g

Gourmet Oat Bowl

Ingredients:

1 full Cup of your preferred grain oat

½ Cup of solidified berries or banana slices

1/8 Cup of toasted nuts

¾ Cup of non fat milk or Soy milk

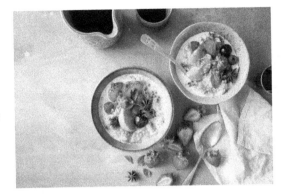

Descriptions:

In a major bowl, put in 1 cup of your preferred entire grain oat with around 30 grams of starches and in any event, 5 grams of fiber. Top with 1/2 cup new or solidified berries or banana cuts and 1/8 cup toasted nuts (almonds, pecans, or walnuts). Shower 3/4 cup nonfat milk or soy milk and mix.

Evaluation:

Starches 48g

Protein 22g

Fiber 15g

French Toast

Ingredients:

1 Egg, 1 Egg white or 2 tablespoons of Egg Substitute

¼ Cup of Non-fat Milk

½ Teaspoon Vanilla Concentrate

¼ Teaspoon ground cinnamon

Wheat Bread

Berries (Crisp or Solidified)

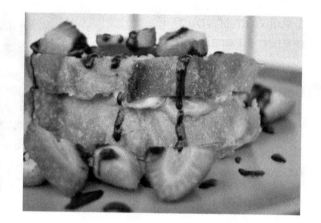

Descriptions:

French toast freezes well, so make some extra on ends of the week to freeze. At that point, microwave it for an exceptional weekday breakfast. For one serving, mix together 1 enormous egg, 1 egg white or 2 tablespoons egg substitute, 1/4 cup nonfat milk or without fat cream, 1/2 teaspoon vanilla concentrate, and 1/4 teaspoon ground cinnamon and blend together. Splash around 3 little or 2 enormous cuts of entire wheat bread in the egg blend. At that point gently dark colored in a non-stick griddle covered with cooking shower. Top with 1/2 cup crisp or solidified berries or other fruits.

Evaluation: Starches 60g - Protein 21g - Fiber 10g

Lunch Recipes

Simple Fish Lunch Plate of mixed greens

Ingredients

6-ounce can stuffed fish

3 Tablespoons of light Italian vinaigrette

Green vegetables

½ Cup of grape or cleaved tomatoes

1/8 cup nuts or olives

2 cups of stuffed spinach leaves

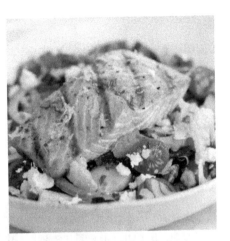

Descriptions

Blend one 6-ounce can water-stuffed fish (depleted) with 3 tablespoons light Italian vinaigrette plate of mixed greens dressing. At that point, include 1/2 cup grape tomatoes or coarsely cleaved tomatoes and 1/8 cup nuts or cut olives. Serve on 2 cups of solidly stuffed spinach leaves. Best enjoyed with an ounce of entire grain wafers.

Nutritional Evaluation

Starches 35g

Protein 54g

Fiber 6g

Grilled Tomato and Cheddar Sandwich With Soup

Ingredients

Wheat Bread

½ ounces reduced fat cheddar

3 cuts vine-aged nursery tomatoes.

Canola Cooking Splash

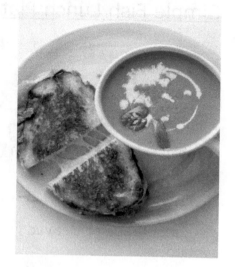

Descriptions

Heat a frying pan covered with cooking splash at average heat. Include a cut of entire wheat bread and top with 1/2 ounces reduced fat cheddar and 3 cuts vine-aged nursery tomatoes. Lay the second bit of entire wheat bread on top and coat the top with canola cooking splash. At the point when the underside is brilliant, flip the sandwich over and delicately dark colored the opposite side. Present with juice or tomato-based soup with around 10 grams of sugars for each 1-cup serving.

Nutritional Evaluation

Starches 60g

Protein 27g

Fiber 8g

Kale and Quinoa Plate of mixed greens with Delicate Bubbled Eggs

Ingredients

1 pack kale, slashed

2 cups destroyed red cabbage

1 cup broccoli slaw

1 chime pepper, cut

2 cups cooked quinoa

2 eggs

1/4 cup disintegrated feta cheddar

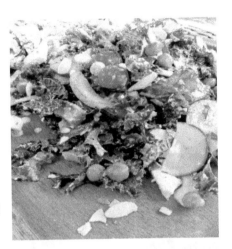

For the dressing

3 tablespoons olive oil

3 tablespoons apple juice vinegar

1 teaspoon dijon mustard

2 cloves garlic, squashed

Descriptions

Heat a huge pot of water to the point of boiling. Delicately pour the eggs into the water with a spoon and turn the warmth to medium-low. Cook for at least 6 minutes and expel with a spoon to a strainer.

Strip any eggs that you'll use later, and keep any outstanding eggs in-shell to strip the prior night use.

To ensure adequate dressing, shake all dressing ingredients in a compact container and refrigerate until it is fully ready to use.

Then, Gap the kale, cabbage, broccoli slaw, and chime peppers into four compartments.

You can easily serve as a plate of mixed greens for lunch, spread 1/4 of the dressing on the veggies and back rub to cover. Include 1/4 of the cooked quinoa, 1 delicate bubbled egg, and 1/4 of the feta. Then just enjoy it!

Nutritional Evaluation

Starches 46g

Protein 24g

Fiber 15g

3-Minute Bean and Cheddar Burrito

Ingredients

Low-carb tortilla

1/3 cup of reduced fat cheddar or Monterey jack

½ cup of refried beans

1 tablespoon without fat acrid cream

1 tablespoon of Salsa

Cleaved Tomato and/or Onions

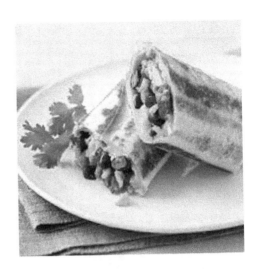

Descriptions

Put a multigrain or low-carb flour tortilla on a paper towel. Microwave on high for around 30 seconds, or until delicate. Sprinkle 1/3 cup destroyed, reduced fat Monterey Jack or cheddar on the highest point of the tortilla. Uniformly spoon 1/2 cup no-fat canned refried beans (or different beans) in the middle, alongside 1 tablespoon without fat acrid cream, 1 tablespoon salsa, and some cleaved green onion or tomato (as wanted). Fold up into a burrito and microwave until hot all through.

Nutritional Evaluation

Starches 50g

Protein 24g

Fiber 10g

Sound Chicken Plate of mixed greens formula

Ingredients

Chicken, destroyed or cut into little pieces

1 celery stalk, cleaved

6-8 grapes, cut

Little bunch pecans, cleaved

Plain Greek or customary yogurt

Dijon mustard

Split pepper

Crisp spinach

Entire wheat pita/bread

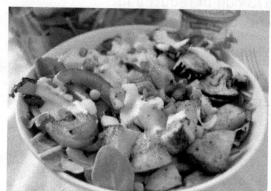

Descriptions

Start with the chicken in a little bowl. Include cleaved celery, grapes, and a little bunch of pecans.

Next, include some split pepper and a spoonful of plain yogurt and a squirt of dijon mustard. Not surprisingly, include around 2 sections yogurt per section of mustard, to taste (Very important, no mayonnaise.)

Blend everything up, place on an entire wheat pita or bread spread with spinach. Sound Chicken Plate of mixed greens formula would likewise be amazing with dried cranberries rather than grapes.

Nutritional Evaluation

Starches 30g - Protein 32g - Fiber 12g

Noon Pasta Plate of mixed greens

Ingredients

1 cup of Cooked Pasta

1 cup of cooked green vegetables (Options: Cabbage, Spinach, broccoli, etc.)

1 ounce scattered part-skim mozzarella (Substitutes include Lean meat, Chicken, or fish)

Sliced tomatoes, onions, and olives

1 tablespoon of walnuts or pecans

2 tablespoons of light vinaigrette

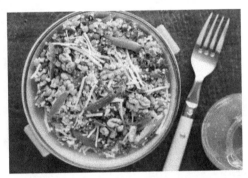

Descriptions

An Extra multigrain pasta from the present dinner can turn out to be tomorrow's lunch! Hurl 1 cup cooked pasta with 1 cup cooked green or cruciferous vegetables of your decision (like broccoli, kale, or cabbage). Include 1 ounce cubed or scattered part-skim mozzarella or 1/2 cup remaining flame broiled fish, chicken, or lean meat, in addition to slashed tomatoes, onions, and cut olives (whenever wanted). Sprinkle 1 tablespoon toasted pine nuts or pecans. Sprinkle on around 2 tablespoons light vinaigrette and hurl. This keeps well in case you're carrying it to work. Store in the cooler.

Nutritional Evaluation

Sugars 54g - Protein 21g -Fiber 10g

Turkey Avocado Wrap

Ingredients

Flatbread or Naan bread

Low-carb tortilla

1 tablespoon of basil

Tomato pesto (sun-dried) or olive tapenade

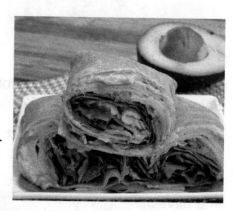

Broiled Turkey

1 ounce of decreased fat provolone or cheddar

4 avocado cuts

Spinach leaves

Tomato slices

Foil

Descriptions

Top a multigrain or low-carb tortilla, flatbread, or naan bread with 1 tablespoon basil, sun-dried tomato pesto, or olive tapenade (accessible in containers). Top with a couple of cuts of broiled turkey, 1 ounce decreased fat provolone (or comparable cheddar), around 4 avocado cuts, a couple of spinach leaves, and some tomato cuts, on choice. Move up and enclose by foil or saran wrap. Chill until prepared to eat.

Nutritional Evaluation

Starches 30g - Protein 32g - Fiber 8g

Dinner Recipes

High-Protein Berry Yogurt Bowl

Ingredients:

1 A cup of Plain nonfat yogurt

1 teaspoon of nectar and ground cinnamon

½ cup of crisp or solidified berries

½ cup of Oat

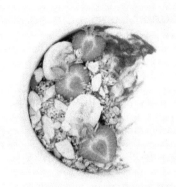

Descriptions:

Put 1 cup plain, nonfat Greek yogurt in a grain bowl. Mix in 1 teaspoon nectar and a sprinkle of ground cinnamon, whenever wanted. Top with 1/2 cup solidified or crisp berries and 1/2 cup entire grain breakfast oat of your decision. (Pick an oat with around 15 grams of sugars and at any rate 5 grams of fiber for every 1/2 cup).

Diabetes Plan

This solid 1,200-calorie weight reduction supper plan for diabetes makes it simple to adjust your glucose.

Nutritional Evaluation

Starches 47g - Protein 22g - Fiber 10g

Vegetarian or Turkey Salsa Bean stew

Ingredients:

1 tablespoon of olive oil

½ pound of dark colored ground lean turkey or 1 pound of cut mushrooms

½ Cleaved Onions

1 teaspoon of Minced garlic

1 cup of Marinara Sauce

15-ounce Can kidney beans

Ground cumin

Pregano

Stew Powder

Descriptions:

In a medium nonstick pan covered with 1 tablespoon extra-virgin olive oil, dark colored 1/2 pound ground lean turkey or 1 pound cut mushrooms with 1/2 cleaved onion and 1 teaspoon minced garlic. Include 1 cup packaged marinara sauce, 1 cup arranged or packaged salsa, 1 15-ounce can dark or kidney beans

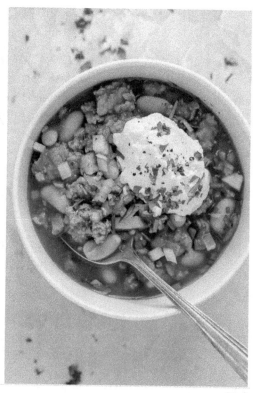

(depleted), in addition to stew powder, oregano, and ground cumin to taste, whenever wanted. Cover and heat to the point of boiling. Lower the warmth and stew for 20 minutes. Makes 3 servings. Present with a cup of organic product plate of mixed greens.

Nutritional Evaluation

Starches 43g

Protein 22g

Fiber 12g

Fruits and Pecan Chicken Dinner Salad

Ingredients:

Skinless Chicken (Choice Size)

3 or 4 Cups of Dull green Lettuce

1 Cup of Crisp or solidified berries

¼ Cup of toasted Walnuts or Pecans

2 tablespoons of Blue Cheddar

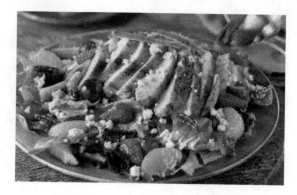

2 tablespoons of light balsamic vinaigrette

Descriptions:

Cut a grilled boneless, skinless chicken into cuts (or use locally acquired pre-cut prepared chicken bosom) and hurl with 3 or 4 cups dull green lettuce, 1 cup crisp or solidified berries or a cut pear or apple, 1/4 cup toasted pecans or walnuts, 2 tablespoons blue cheddar, and 2 tablespoons light balsamic or raspberry vinaigrette.

Nutritional Evaluation

Starches 27g

Protein 37g

Fiber 12g

Teriyaki Salmon Dinner (Another choice of Fish or skinless chicken is welcomed)

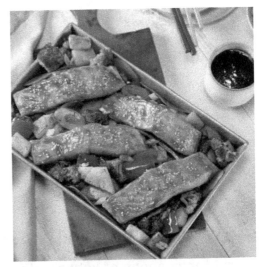

Ingredients

Dark Colored Rice

Skinless Chicken

Salmon Filets

Teriyaki Sauce

Vegetables

Descriptions:

Cook steamed dark colored rice (accessible in the food section in some supermarkets). While it cooks, heat the grill of your broiler or toaster-stove. Line a pie plate with foil and spot salmon filets on top. Sprinkle each filet with 2 teaspoons packaged teriyaki sauce. Sear around 6 creeps from the oven for around 4 minutes. Flip the fish, spread 1 tablespoon teriyaki sauce over each piece, and sear until the fish is cooked through. Present with 3/4 cup steamed dark colored rice and 1 cup steamed green or cruciferous vegetables per serving.

Nutritional Evaluation:

Starches 42g

Protein 29g

Fiber 5g

Mushroom Spaghetti Dinner

Ingredients

Spaghetti

1 Cup cut of Mushrooms

½ teaspoons of Olive oil per pot

¾ cup of marinara sauce

2 cups of Spinach or Romaine lettuce

¼ cup of garbanzo or kidney beans

Vegetable slices like Carrots, cucumber, so on

1 or 2 tablespoons of light vinaigrette

Descriptions

Bubble entire grain spaghetti as per bundle bearings. While it cooks, sauté 1 cup cut mushrooms (any sort) and 1/2 teaspoons olive oil for each in a medium non-stick pot. Pour in 3/4 cup marinara sauce for every individual, spread, and heat to the point of boiling. Lessen warmth to a stew and cook for 10 minutes. Serve around 1 cup of the mushroom

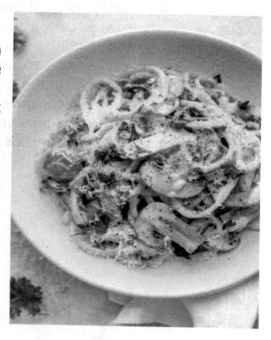

marinara with 3/4 cup cooked pasta. Present with a nursery serving of mixed greens: Hurl 2 cups spinach or romaine lettuce, 1/4 cup kidney or garbanzo beans, a couple of olives, and arranged vegetables, such as cucumber and carrot slices with a tablespoon or two of light vinaigrette.

Evaluation:

Starches 60g

Protein18g

Fiber 9g

Salmon is a diabetes superfood.

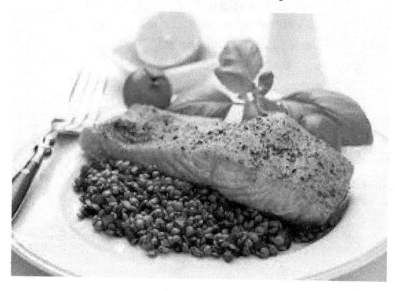

Type 2 diabetes includes issues getting enough glucose into the cells. At the point when the sugar can't get where it should be, it prompts raised glucose levels in the circulation system, which can prompt complexities, for example, kidney, nerve, and eye harm, and cardiovascular ailment.

Nourishments to eat for a sort 2 diabetic eating regimen supper plan incorporate complex sugars, for example, darker rice, entire wheat, quinoa, cereal, organic products, vegetables, beans, and lentils. Nourishments to maintain a strategic distance from incorporate straightforward starches, which are handled, for example, sugar, pasta, white bread, flour, and treats, cakes.

Nourishments with a low glycemic load (list) just aim an unassuming ascent in glucose and are better decisions for individuals with diabetes. Great glycemic control can help in forestalling long haul difficulties of type 2 diabetes.

Fats don't have a lot of an immediate impact on glucose, yet they can be helpful in easing back the ingestion of starches.

Protein furnishes relentless vitality with little impact on glucose. It keeps glucose stable and can help with sugar desires and feeling full in the wake of eating. Protein-stuffed nourishments to eat incorporate beans, vegetables, eggs, fish, dairy, peas, tofu, and lean meats and poultry.

Five diabetes "superfoods" to eat incorporate chia seeds, wild salmon, white balsamic vinegar, cinnamon, and lentils.

Solid diabetes dinner plans incorporate a lot of vegetables and restricted prepared sugars and red meat.

Diet suggestions for individuals with type 2 diabetes incorporate a veggie lover or vegetarian diet, the American Diabetes Affiliation diet (which additionally underscores work out), the Paleo Diet, and the Mediterranean eating routine.

Rules on what to eat for individuals with type 2 diabetes incorporate eating low glycemic load starches, essentially from vegetables, and devouring fats and proteins for the most part from plant sources.

What to not to eat in the event that you have type 2 diabetes: soft drinks (standard and diet), refined sugars, handled starches, trans fats, high-fat creature items, high-fat dairy items, high fructose corn syrup, fake sugars, and any exceptionally prepared nourishments.

What is a Paleo Diet?

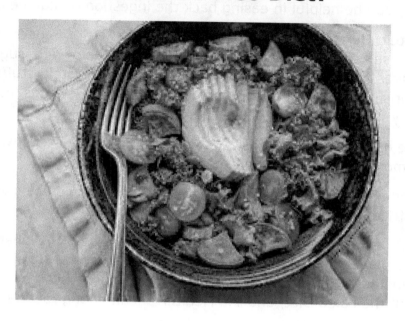

Paleolithic weight control plans incorporate a reasonable measure of protein and have increased a great deal of consideration as of late. The hypothesis behind this dietary example is that our hereditary foundation has not developed to meet our cutting edge way of life of calorically thick accommodation nourishments and restricted movement, and that coming back to a tracker gatherer method for eating will work better with human physiology. This has been considered in a couple of little preliminaries, and it seems valuable for individuals with type 2 diabetes.

The Paleolithic eating routine depends on:
· Lean meat
· Fish, natural product
· Verdant and cruciferous vegetables
· Root vegetables
· Eggs

· Nuts

The Paleolithic eating routine rejects:
· Dairy items
· Grains of different sorts
· Beans
· Refined fats
· Sugar
· Sweet
· Sodas
· Brew
· Any additional option of salt

The Paleo Diet doesn't indicate macronutrient balance or caloric admission objectives.

As a general rule, when individuals in an examination followed the Paleolithic eating regimen, it turned out the eating routine was lower in all-out vitality, vitality thickness, starches, dietary glycemic load, fiber, soaked unsaturated fats, and calcium; yet higher in unsaturated fats (great fats), dietary cholesterol, and a few nutrients and minerals. Research likewise exhibits that individuals with diabetes are less hungry, have progressively stable glucose, and feel better with lower starch eats fewer carbs.

What is the Mediterranean eating routine?

The Mediterranean eating regimen is high in vegetables. This alludes to the actual Mediterranean example generally followed in the south of Italy and Greece, not "Assimilated Italian," which is overwhelming in pasta and bread. The Mediterranean example incorporates:

- Heaps of new vegetables
- Some organic product
- Plant-fats, for example, olive oil
- Avocados and nuts
- Fish, for example, sardines
- Some wine
- Intermittent meat and dairy

This example of eating is supplement thick, which means you get numerous nutrients, minerals, and other empowering supplements for each calorie devoured. An exceptionally enormous late examination exhibited that two renditions of the Mediterranean eating routine improved diabetes control, including better glucose and more weight reduction. The two versions of the Mediterranean eating routine that were considered underscored either increasingly nuts or progressively olive oil. Since both were gainful, a presence of mind way to deal with embracing the Mediterranean eating regimen would incorporate both of these. For instance, sprinkle cleaved almonds on green beans or shower zucchini with olive oil, oregano, and hemp seeds.

Prescribed nourishments
Make the most of your calories with these nutritious nourishments. Pick sound starches, fiber-rich nourishments, fish, and "great" fats.
Solid starches
During assimilation, sugars (straightforward carbs) and carbohydrates (complex carbohydrates) separate into blood glucose. Concentrate on stable starches, for example,

- Organic products
- Vegetables
- Entire grains

· Vegetables, for example, beans, and peas
· Low-fat dairy items, for example, milk and cheddar
· Maintain a strategic distance from fewer sound starches, for instance, nourishments or beverages with included fats, sugars, and sodium.
· Fiber-rich nourishments
Dietary fiber incorporates all pieces of plant nourishments that your body can't process or retain. Fiber directs how your body processes and assists control with blooding sugar levels. Nourishments high in fiber include:
· Vegetables
· Organic products
· Nuts
· Vegetables, for example, beans and peas
· Entire grains
· Heart-solid fish

Eat heart-solid fish, in any event, two times every week. Fish, for example, salmon, mackerel, fish, and sardines, are wealthy in omega-3 unsaturated fats, which may forestall coronary illness.
Maintain a strategic distance from seared fish and fish with significant levels of mercury, for example, ruler mackerel.
'Great' fats
Nourishments containing monounsaturated and polyunsaturated fats can help bring down your cholesterol levels. These include:
- Avocados
- Nuts
- Canola, olive and nut oils
- In any case, don't try too hard, as all fats are high in calories.
A dietitian can show you how to gauge nourishment divides and become an informed peruser of nourishment

names. The person can likewise show you how to give extraordinary consideration to serving size and starch content.

In case you're taking insulin, a dietitian can show you how to include the measure of starches in every dinner or nibble and change your insulin portion as needs are.

Pick your nourishments

A dietitian may prescribe you pick explicit nourishments to assist you with arranging dinners and bites. You can choose various nourishments from records, including classes, for example, sugars, proteins, and fats.

One serving in a class is known as a "decision." A nourishment decision has about a similar measure of sugars, protein, fat, and calories — and a similar impact on your blood glucose — as a serving of each other nourishment in that equivalent classification. For instance, the starch, foods grown from the ground list incorporates decisions that are 12 to 15 grams of sugars.

One Week Dieting Plan

When arranging dinner, consider your size and movement level. The accompanying menu is customized for somebody who needs 1,200 to 1,600 calories every day.

Breakfast. Entire wheat bread (1 medium cut) with 2 teaspoons jam, 1/2 cup destroyed wheat grain with some 1 percent low-fat milk, a bit of organic product, espresso

Lunch. Broil hamburger sandwich on wheat bread with lettuce, low-fat American cheddar, tomato and mayonnaise, a medium apple, water

Supper. Salmon, 1/2 teaspoons vegetable oil, little prepared potato, 1/2 cup carrots, 1/2 cup green beans, medium white supper roll, unsweetened frosted tea, milk

Bite. 2 1/2 cups popcorn with 1/2 teaspoons margarine

Eating well with diabetes is simple and delicious with this diabetes diet plan. The straightforward suppers and bites that make this arrangement so essential and sensible to follow include the best nourishments for diabetes, similar to complex starches (think entire grains and new products of the soil), lean protein, and solid fats. The carbohydrates are offset during each time with every feast containing 2-3 carb servings (30-45 grams of sugars) and each tidbit providing around 1 carb serving (15 grams of carbs). To help prevent your glucose from spiking too high too rapidly, we restricted refined starches (like white bread, white pasta, and white rice) and have likewise eliminated immersed fats and sodium, which can contrarily affect your wellbeing on the off chance that you eat excessively.

What we unquestionably didn't hold back on is season. The dinners and snacks in this eating routine arrangement highlight crisp fixings and a lot of herbs and flavors that include season without including additional sodium. Eating with diabetes shouldn't be troublesome— pick an assortment of nutritious nourishments, as we do in this eating routine dinner plan, and include every day practice for a sound and maintainable way to deal with overseeing diabetes

See all our sound dinner plans for diabetes, and don't miss our assortment of delectable diabetes-accommodating plans.

Prep the Chipotle-Lime Cauliflower Taco Bowls and store in a water/air proof compartment to have like an instant lunch on Days 2 through 5.

Make 5 servings of the Cinnamon Roll Medium-term Oats and store in sealed cotainers to have as get and-go morning meals on Days 2 through 6.

Start the Moderate Cooker Vegetable Soup early enough on Day 1 with the goal that it's prepared before supper time.

One Week Dieting Plan

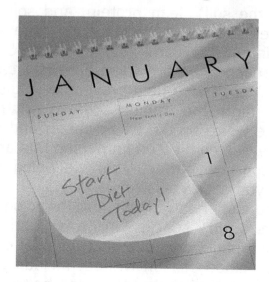

When arranging dinner, consider your size and movement level. The accompanying menu is customized for somebody who needs 1,200 to 1,600 calories every day.

Breakfast: Entire wheat bread (1 medium cut) with 2 teaspoons jam, 1/2 cup destroyed wheat grain with some 1 percent low-fat milk, a bit of organic product, espresso

Lunch: Broil hamburger sandwich on wheat bread with lettuce, low-fat American cheddar, tomato and mayonnaise, a medium apple, water

Dinner: Salmon, 1/2 teaspoons vegetable oil, little prepared potato, 1/2 cup carrots, 1/2 cup green beans,

medium white supper roll, unsweetened frosted tea, milk
Bite. 2 1/2 cups popcorn with 1/2 teaspoons margarine

Eating well with diabetes is simple and delicious with this diabetes diet plan. The straightforward suppers and bites that make this arrangement so essential and sensible to follow include the best nourishments for diabetes, similar to complex starches (think entire grains and new products of the soil), lean protein, and solid fats. The carbohydrates are offset during each time with every feast containing 2-3 carb servings (30-45 grams of sugars) and each tidbit providing around 1 carb serving (15 grams of carbs).

To help prevent your glucose from spiking too high too rapidly, we restricted refined starches (like white bread, white pasta, and white rice) and have likewise eliminated immersed fats and sodium, which can contrarily affect your wellbeing on the off chance that you eat excessively.

What we unquestionably didn't hold back on is season. The dinners and snacks in this eating routine arrangement highlight crisp fixings and a lot of herbs and flavors that include season without including additional sodium. Eating with diabetes shouldn't be troublesome— pick an assortment of nutritious nourishments, as we do in this eating routine dinner plan, and include every day practice for a sound and maintainable way to deal with overseeing diabetes

See all our sound dinner plans for diabetes, and don't miss our assortment of delectable diabetes-accommodating plans.

Prep the Chipotle-Lime Cauliflower Taco Bowls and store in a water/air proof compartment to have like an instant lunch on Days 2 through 5.

Make 5 servings of the Cinnamon Roll Medium-term Oats and store in sealed cotainers to have as get and-go morning meals on Days 2 through 6.

Start the Moderate Cooker Vegetable Soup early enough on Day 1 with the goal that it's prepared before supper time.

Day 1

Morning (281 calories, 33 g sugars)

Ingredients
1 serving Bagel Avocado Toast
1/2 cup blueberries
1/2 nonfat plain Greek yogurt
10 pistachios

Afternoon (325 calories, 40 g sugars)

1 serving Veggie and Hummus Sandwich
1 medium apple, cut and sprinkled with cinnamon

Evening (428 calories, 47 g sugars)

2 cups Moderate Cooker Vegetable Soup beat with 2 Tablespoons of scattered Parmesan cheddar
1 cut entire wheat bread, toasted and sprinkled with 2 tablespoons of olive oil

Tip: Spare at least 2 cups each of the Moderate Cooker Vegetable Soup and store in a water/air proof holder for Day 6 and 7.

Overall Nutrition Evaluation:

Calories 1,195
Protein 54g
Starches 148g
Fiber 37g
Sugar 49g
Healthy Fat 49g
Saturated fat 9g
Sodium 1,924mg

Day 2

Morning (Calories 276, Starches 43g)

1 serving Cinnamon Roll Medium-term Oats
1/2 cup raspberries
1 Tbsp. cleaved walnuts
5 different fruits

Afternoon (Calories 344, Sugars 47g)

1 serving Chipotle-Lime Cauliflower Taco Bowls
1 medium apple, cut and sprinkled with cinnamon

Evening (Calories 411, Sugars 41g)

2 1/2 cups Lentil and Cooked Vegetable Serving of mixed greens with Green Goddess Dressing beat with 1/2 cup bread garnishes

Overall Nutrition Evaluation:

Calories 1,204
Protein 37g
Starches 176g
Fiber40g
Sugar 61g
Fat 45g

Soaked fat 8g
Sodium 1,638 mg

Day 3

*Morning (*Calories 276, Starches 43g)

1 serving Cinnamon Roll Medium-term Oats
1/2 cup raspberries
1 Tbsp. hacked walnuts
1 medium plum

Afternoon (Calories 344, Starches 47g)

1 serving Chipotle-Lime Cauliflower Taco Bowls or Turkey sandwich on entire wheat with cut veggies
1 medium orange

Evening (Calories 483, Sugars 53g)

1/3 cups Chicken Frankfurter and Peppers
1/2 cup cooked darker rice hurled with 1/2 tsp. every olive oil and no-salt-included Italian flavoring
2 cups blended greens beat with 2 Tbsp. Italian vinaigrette dressing*

*When purchasing premade serving of mixed greens dressings, search for one made without included sugars. Furthermore, pick one made with olive oil or canola oil.

Make Ahead Tip: Cook an additional 1/2 cup of dark colored rice to have for Dinner on Day 7. You can substitute dark colored rice for the farro in the supper formula for Day 4. On the off chance that you decide to do as such, cook an additional 2 cups of rice today to spare yourself time tomorrow.

Overall Nutrition Evaluation:

Calories 1,195

Protein 45g

Starches 166g

Fiber 35g

Sugar 54g

Fat 44g

Saturated fat, 9g

Sodium 1,678mg

Day 4

Morning (Calories 276, starches 43g)

1 serving Cinnamon Roll Medium-term Oats
1/2 cup raspberries
1 Tbsp. slashed walnuts
15 fruits

Afternoon (Calories 344, sugars 47g)

1 serving Chipotle-Lime Cauliflower Taco Bowls or Turkey
bean stew with diminished fat cheddar
1 medium orange

Evening (Calories 450, sugars 41g)

1 serving Lemon-Herb Salmon with Caponata and Farro*

*Don't have farro? You can substitute another entire grain
you have close by, similar to dark colored rice.

Overall Nutrition Evaluation:

Calories 1,209
Protein 58g
Starches 166g
Fiber 36g
Sugar 60g
Fat 40g
Immersed fat 7g
Sodium 1,422mg

Day 5

Morning (Calories 276, Starches 43g)

1 serving Cinnamon Roll Medium-term Oats or Fruit smoothie
made with low-fat milk, yogurt, and chia seeds
(discretionary)
1/2 cup raspberries
1 Tablespoon slashed walnuts
1 plum

Afternoon (344 calories, 47 g sugars)
1 serving Chipotle-Lime Cauliflower Taco Bowls
P.M. Bite (103 calories, 26 g starches)
20 fruits

Evening (457 calories, 36 g starches)

1 serving Spaghetti Squash and Meatballs or Tofu and veggie
pan sear over darker rice

1/2 cups blended greens bested with 1 Tablespoon. Italian
vinaigrette dressing

Overall Nutrition Evaluation:

Calories 1,211
Protein 54g
Starches 160g
Fiber 36g

Sugar 63g
Fat 44g
Immersed fat 9g
Sodium 1,635mg

Day 6

Morning (Calories 276, Starches 43g)

1 serving Cinnamon Roll Medium-Size Oats or Veggie omelet (1 entire egg in addition to 2 egg whites), bested with decreased fat cheddar, in addition, Fruits such are Orange or Apples

1/2 cup raspberries
1 Tablespoon of cleaved walnuts
25 fruits

Afternoon (calories 275, Starches 36g)

2 cups Moderate Cooker Vegetable Soup bested with 2 Tbsp. destroyed Parmesan cheddar
1 medium orange

Evening (calories 464, Starches 53g)

1 serving Apple-Coated Chicken with Spinach
1/2 cup Steamed Butternut Squash hurled with 1 tablespoon of extra-virgin olive oil, 1/2 tablespoon of thyme, and a little pinch of salt and pepper.

Overall Nutrition Evaluation:

Calories 1,206
Protein 59g
Starches 180g
Absolute fiber 33g
Sugar 87g
Fat 35g,

6g soaked fat
Sodium 2,288mg

Day 7

Morning (Calories 349, Starches 59g)

2 Blueberry-Walnut Flapjacks
1/2 cup blueberries, new or solidified
1 Tbsp. maple syrup
1 medium orange

Afternoon (Calories 254, Starches 35g)

2 cups Moderate Cooker Vegetable Soup bested with 1 Tbsp. destroyed Parmesan cheddar or A Plate of mixed greens (dull lettuce or verdant greens) bested with chicken bosom and chickpeas with olive oil and vinegar dressing

1 medium apple

Evening (Calories 444, Starches 48g)

1 serving Mushroom-Sauced Pork Cleaves or Well grilled salmon, steamed broccoli, and quinoa
1/2 cup cooked dark colored rice
3/4 cup Cooked Brussels Sprouts with Sun-Dried Tomato Pesto

Tip: Today, around evening time's supper is a moderate cooker formula. Ensure you start it early enough in the day that it will be prepared in time for supper.

Overall Nutrition Evaluation:

Calories 1,203
 Protein 59g,
Starches 183g

Fiber29g
Sugar 77g
Fat 31g
Saturated fat 6g
Sodium 1,775mg

Fundamentally, there's no size-fits-all diabetes diet, yet seeing how to settle on keen nourishment decisions is basic for keeping glucose in a solid range. A fantastic diabetes diet comprises of all the key nutrition classes, including natural products, veggies, solid fat, and protein. Living great with diabetes implies accepting your drug as recommended, overseeing pressure, practicing normally, and similarly significant, realizing what nourishments are acceptable and awful for keeping your glucose levels in a solid range. In the event that you've recently been determined to have type 2 diabetes, the possibility of surrendering the nourishments you love may appear to be overwhelming or in any event, annihilating. In any case, you might be mitigated to realize that a decent eating routine for type 2 diabetes isn't as mind boggling or strange as you would anticipate.

How Cutting Carbs Can Assist You With balancing out Unequal Glucose Levels That Outcome From Diabetes

The best game-plan is dealing with the measure of sugars you eat. "Albeit singular sugar objectives will shift dependent on age, action level, drug, and individual insulin obstruction levels, it's basic to abstain from having an excessive number of starches in a single sitting," says Palinski-Swim. For reference, on the off chance that you have prediabetes or type

2 diabetes and don't take medicine, top carbs to close to 60 grams (g) per supper (four sugar servings).

The best wellsprings of starches for somebody with diabetes are fiber-rich sources from entire nourishments, which can help improve glucose control. These incorporate natural products, vegetables, sans fat or low-fat dairy, and entire grains. Farthest point sugar and refined grains, similar to white bread and pasta.

What Are the Best Kinds of Proteins While taking care of Type 2 Diabetes?

One-fourth of your plate ought to contain a wellspring of lean protein, which incorporates meat, skinless poultry, fish, diminished fat cheddar, eggs, and vegan sources, similar to beans and tofu. Appreciate these diabetes-accommodating choices:

- Beans, including dark or kidney beans
- Hummus
- Lentils
- Edamame
- Nut spread
- Tofu
- Fish, for example, fish, sardines, or salmon
- Skinless poultry
- Eggs
- Low-fat or without fat curds
- Decreased fat cheddar or customary cheddar in limited quantities
- Lean meat, similar to sirloin or tenderloin

Fat isn't the adversary, regardless of whether you have diabetes! The key is having the option to tell undesirable fats from sound fats and appreciating them with some restraint, as all fats are high in calories.

In any case, type matters more than sum: Expect to restrain soaked fat from closing to 10 percent of all out calories, Palinski-Swim exhorts.

Consider choosing these wellsprings of solid fat, per the American Diabetes Affiliation (ADA):

- Avocado
- Oils, including canola, corn, and safflower
- Nuts, for example, almonds, peanuts, and pecans
- Olive oil
- Seeds, including sesame, pumpkin, and sunflower

What Are the Best Wellsprings of Dairy When You Have Type 2 Diabetes?

The objective with dairy is to pick sources that are nonfat or low-fat (1 percent) to save money on soaked fat. Likewise, recall that while these sources offer protein, they are additionally another wellspring of carbs, so you have to figure them your carb portion.

- Nonfat or 1 percent milk
- Nonfat or low-fat plain yogurt (just as Greek yogurt)
- Nonfat or low-fat curds
- Nondairy milk, similar to soy milk or almond milk
- Diminished fat cheddar

Try not to fear grains either — they're an extraordinary wellspring of heart-sound fiber. Mean to make in any event half of your grain consumption entire grains. Here are some incredible alternatives:

- Antiquated or steel-cut oats
- 100 percent entire wheat bread, wraps, or tortillas

- Entire grain oat (without included sugar)
- Quinoa
- Dark colored rice
- Farro
- Entire grain pasta
- Grain
- Bulgur
- Millet
- Wild rice

What Are the Most beneficial Toppings for Overseeing Type 2 Diabetes?

Sugar stows away in numerous fixings, similar to ketchup, bar-b-que sauce, and marinades. Continuously read the mark, and pick the lower-sugar alternative that best fits in with your eating routine and objectives. Here are a couple of sauces recommended by the ADA that lift the kind of nourishments without causing a sugar over-burden.

- Mustard (Dijon or entire grain)
- Salsa
- Olive oil
- Vinegar, including balsamic, red or white wine, or apple juice assortments
- Flavors and herbs
- Light serving of mixed greens dressing (without included sugar)
- Hot sauce
- Hummus

The Best nutrition to Eat Routinely in the event that You Are Living With Type 2 Diabetes

Certain nourishments are viewed as staples in a sort 2 diabetes diet. These are nourishments that are known to assist control with blooding sugar and advance a sound weight. They include:

Fiber-rich leafy foods vegetables, for example, apples and broccoli

Lean wellsprings of protein, for example, boneless, skinless chicken, turkey, and greasy fish, similar to salmon

Sound fats, for example, nutty spread, nuts, and avocado (with some restraint)

Entire grains, like quinoa and grain

Nonfat or low-fat dairy, similar to milk and plain yogurt

The Top Nourishments to Constrain or Maintain a strategic distance from on the off chance that You Have Type 2 Diabetes

Moreover, certain nourishments are known to toss glucose levels askew and advance unfortunate weight gain. Nourishments that ought to be constrained or stayed away from on the off chance that you have type 2 diabetes include:

- Chips
- Treats
- Cake
- White bread and pasta
- Canned soups, which are high in sodium
- Microwaveable suppers, which are likewise high in sodium
- Treat

- Wellsprings of immersed fat, similar to bacon or greasy cuts of meat

Hints for Building a Decent Diabetes Plan

Your first stop ought to associate with an enlisted dietitian who is a guaranteed diabetes teacher — scan for one close to you at EatRight.org — and your essential specialist to make sense of what number of starches you ought to eat per supper dependent on your individual needs, says Palinski-Swim. From that point, follow this means:

Know "like" nourishments. Utilize a diabetes trade list, which discloses to you how nourishments look at as far as their starch content. For example, 1 apple and ½ cup fruit purée both contain around 15 g of carbs. Or figure out how to tally starches — an arrangement of considering sugars in nourishments in 15 g units. This will assist you with deciding legitimate bits.

Utilize the Make Your Plate apparatus. At the point when you're simply beginning, it's useful to imagine precisely what your plate ought to resemble. The ADA has a Make Your Plate apparatus that will help massively. With enough practice, this will turn out to be natural. They suggest filling a large portion of your plate with nonstarchy vegetables (broccoli, spinach, tomatoes), one-quarter with grains (ideally entire) or dull nourishments (sweet potato, plantain), and another quarter with lean protein (beans, fish, skinless chicken).

Top it off. A shrewd expansion to the supper is a serving of organic products or nonfat or low-fat dairy. Drink water or unsweetened tea or espresso.

Season right. Utilizing salt on your nourishments is fine (and upgrades the flavor), however observe the amount you include. Focus on under 2,300 mg of sodium for each day (and under 1,500 mg day by day on the off chance that you have coronary illness). Utilizing dried herbs and flavors is another approach to add without sodium flavor to nourishments for no calories.

It can appear to be difficult to explore a menu when you're eating out, yet it's certainly feasible. Make the most of your time with companions and eat delectable nourishment with these rules from Palinski-Swim:

Have an application before you leave. It's enticing to "set aside" calories for the duration of the day to help plan for a night out, however that approach can reverse discharge. You'll be hungry when you arrive and less inclined to settle on a sound decision when you request. Eat a little, solid nibble before you go, similar to certain nuts or a low-fat plain yogurt. "This can assist decline with wanting and forestall gorging" she says.

Imagine your plate. In a perfect world, your plate should look fundamentally the same as how it does at home — with a few little changes: 1/2 vegetables (steamed if conceivable), 1/4 lean protein, and 1/4 entire grains. "You need to be mindful so as not to eat such a large number of carbs at one sitting, and keep away from dinners pressed with soaked fat," says Palinski-Swim.

Taste shrewd. Liquor stirs your hunger, so in the event that you do have liquor (make a point to converse with your primary care physician first in case you're taking drugs), do as such close to the finish of the feast. Limit it to one glass.

Step by step instructions to Discover Additional Assistance Building a Sort 2 Diabetes-Accommodating Eating routine

On the off chance that you have diabetes, you definitely know how accommodating having a solid emotionally supportive network can be. In any case, that system ought to reach out past simply your loved ones. That is the place that enrolled dietitian or ensured diabetes instructor becomes an integral factor.

"Diabetes is an extremely singular illness. Contingent upon factors like your age, movement level, insulin opposition, and prescription, your dietary objectives and sugar objectives can fluctuate incredibly," Palinski-Swim clarifies.

An expert who knows nourishment and diabetes all around can assist you with making an arrangement that meets your objectives for weight reduction and glucose levels, yet isn't prohibitive to such an extent that you can't make the most of your preferred food sources, she includes.

Your eating routine is one of the fundamental mainstays of good diabetes control. "What you eat can help or prevent insulin obstruction," says Palinski-Swim.

While it appears as though there is a ton to recall, the essential principles come down to straightforward, nutritious eating.

At last, you can slice through the commotion by considering a couple of things when you plunk down to eat: Focus on "a well-adjusted eating routine restricted in basic sugars and wealthy in entire plant-based nourishments, for example, vegetables and organic product, alongside lean proteins, entire grains, and sound, plant-based fats," she says.

Recollect that and you don't have to keep a huge amount of rules — in any event, when you have type 2 diabetes.

Three eating regimen methodologies to help anybody determined to have prediabetes or type 2 diabetes become more astute about controlling your glucose, diminish regular complexities, and accomplish a solid weight.

An analysis of type 2 diabetes—or even prediabetes—normally implies the specialist has recommended that you roll out certain improvements to your eating regimen or the eating routine of somebody you care for. This is a decent time to get more astute about how you are eating all the time.

Luckily, following a diabetes diet doesn't mean surrendering the delight of eating or maintaining a strategic distance from your preferred nourishments and extraordinary family suppers. You can even now appreciate "pizza night," praise birthday celebrations and commemorations, and participate in occasion suppers and excursion eating. This is increasingly about your normal day by day nourishment decisions and supper arranging.

Arranging a tasty feast that meets the objectives of a diabetes diet.

Utilize the four segments of a plate as a guide when arranging solid suppers for somebody with diabetes.

Eating to beat diabetes is considerably more about making insightful nourishment alterations than it is about forswearing and hardship. A superior method to take a gander at an eating routine when you have diabetes is one that causes you build up another typical with regards to your dietary patterns and nourishment choices.

Receiving a Diabetes Diet Plan for Long haul Wellbeing

By turning into more smart about the impact that nourishments, particularly carbs, can have on your glucose, you will need to know how and for what reason to alter your nourishment decisions; you can feel such a great amount of better all the while.

It might facilitate your psyche to realize you will have the option to consolidate your preferred nourishments into a sound eating regimen while being aware of your diabetes diet objectives (eg, solid weight, relentless blood glucose levels, great circulatory strain). For some individuals, in any event at first, this may appear to be more diligently than it ought to be and that is reasonable; all things considered, it can appear to be extremely, testing to change current dietary patterns and locate the correct nourishment musicality to accommodate your way of life.

You don't need to go only it—Look for guidance from an enlisted dietitian (RD) or guaranteed diabetes teacher (CDE) who has the correct preparing to assist you with concocting an individualized supper plan that will assist you with meeting your self-administration objectives, get the nourishment you need, and give you how you can consolidate a portion of your preferred food sources into your eating routine so you keep on appreciating eating. Ideally, your PCP has somebody in the group, however on the off chance that not, call your wellbeing safety net provider to request the names of a couple in-arrange RD/CDEs.

There are likewise virtual instructing programs that show up extremely powerful; this implies you can get individualized dietary direction at home or at work. Most medical coverage organizations will take care of the expense of diabetic eating routine directing so approach your primary care physician for a medicine so cost doesn't keep you down.

"While changing your eating routine can be befuddling and overpowering from the outset, examine shows that creation sound way of life decisions can assist you with dealing with your glucose levels for the time being and may even forestall a considerable lot of the long haul wellbeing difficulties related with diabetes," says Lori Zanini, RD, CDE, and writer of The Diabetes Cookbook and Feast Plan for the Recently Analyzed.

In spite of the fact that you can remember most nourishments for a diabetic eating routine, you do need to give most consideration to especially to the sorts of starches you pick so as to forestall spikes, or unfortunate increments, in your glucose.

Nourishments high in straightforward starches—for the most part from included sugars (ie, natural sweetener, dark colored sugar, maple syrup, nectar) and refined grains (particularly white flour and white rice)— as nourishments containing these fixings will cause your glucose levels to rise more rapidly than nourishments that contain fiber, for example, 100% entire wheat and oats.

"Everybody is extraordinary and, at last, you know best how your body reacts to various kinds of nourishments, so you may need to make singular modifications when cooking at home, eating out, or going to festivities," Ms. Zanini calls attention to. "You may locate that some prepared, high-carb nourishments, similar to business breakfast grains and plain white rice, are simply unreasonably "spiky" for you and it's ideal to avoid them and find sensible substitutes."

There are various kinds of diabetes, decided for the most part by your body's capacity to create and utilize insulin—the hormone essential for getting sugar out of your blood and into your cells where it is utilized to deliver vitality.

The indications of a wide range of diabetes are comparative, so the means you have to take to control your glucose continue as before. Your eating routine assumes a basic job in dealing with your diabetes by keeping glucose levels stable all through your lifetime. You are in charge of what you eat, so this is one zone you can and ought to figure out how to oversee shrewdly.

For individuals with type 2 diabetes, your pancreas delivers a lot of insulin that isn't detected by the cells so your body can't appropriately utilize the insulin you make. For the most part, type 2 diabetes can be controlled well with way of life changes—especially moving from handled carbs to high fiber nourishments, and strolling day by day—varying with the expansion of medication.

"A few people with type 2 diabetes may likewise need to start taking insulin sooner or later," says Sandra Arevalo, MPH, RD, CDE, a diabetes master and representative with the Foundation of Sustenance and Dietetics. "It can rely upon your age and your individual capacity to control your glucose with diet and exercise." Be that as it may, when type 2 diabetes is discovered early enough and weight reduction is accomplished, as a rule, insulin is rarely required.

A determination of prediabetes implies that your glucose levels are marginally over the typical range on the grounds that your body is never again reacting to insulin viably, yet not yet sufficiently high for a finding of type 2 diabetes.

By making a few changes in accordance with your flow nourishment designs, and expanding your degree of physical movement, it is conceivable, even likely, that you can forestall or defer the movement to diabetes, just as lessen your danger of coronary illness and different difficulties related with inadequately controlled diabetes.

"You don't really need to follow a severe nourishment routine and evade a wide range of nourishments when you're determined to have diabetes or prediabetes," Ms. Arevalo includes. "You simply need to figure out how to consolidate various sorts of nourishments in a similar dinner and measure those food sources so you eat fitting sums."

Joining nourishments, by consolidating a carb with either protein or some fat, is the best stunt for controlling glucose, and keeping it relentless. The nourishment parcels, as you may expect, have more to do with meeting your vitality needs however not expending abundance calories, which get put away as fat, prompting bothersome weight gain.

Three Diabetes Diet Procedures: Essential Rules for Individuals with Diabetes

Finding your way to a sound eating routine can decrease the dangers related with diabetes. There are three principle objectives, as per the American Diabetes Affiliation (ADA), so following these demonstrated systems will push you to:

1. Accomplish a sound body weight: Weight file (BMI) utilizes your tallness and weight to decide how a lot of muscle versus fat you convey. A BMI of 18.5 to 25 is viewed as a sound weight territory with a solid measure of muscle versus fat. Another measure: abdomen circuit (WC) is considered by numerous individuals to be a superior proportion of overabundance stomach muscle versus fat. A midsection boundary—more noteworthy than 40 creeps for men, or more 35 crawls in ladies—has been appeared to expand the danger of creating medical issues, for example, type 2 diabetes, coronary illness, and hypertension.

The closer you are to a sound body weight or if nothing else a satisfactory midriff outline, the more probable you will have the option to control and, conceivably turn around your dangers of diabetes.

"Try not to get overpowered by contemplating how a lot of all out weight you need to lose," Ms. Arevalo exhorts. "Studies have indicated that losing only 5-10% of your body weight will essentially improve your glucose levels just as your cardiovascular wellbeing so set transient objectives of losing only 5-10 pounds to begin."

2. Achieve typical lab results. Your doctor will work with you to set up singular objectives for blood glucose, blood cholesterol, and circulatory strain. Standard testing will help guarantee that your eating regimen plan, practice procedures

and drug, if vital, are for the most part cooperating to keep your glucose, lipids, circulatory strain, and your body weight, in solid reaches.

3. Maintain a strategic distance from future inconveniences. Way of life changes, including acclimations to your eating regimen and the expansion of customary physical action (regardless of whether just a 30 brief every day walk), can decrease your danger of creating coronary illness, kidney malady, nerve harm, stroke, visual impairment, and other long haul medical issues that can usually happen in individuals with diabetes.

Embracing a Diet Plan for Diabetes

As indicated by the American Diabetes Affiliation (ADA), a Mediterranean-style diet, a plant-based eating routine, and an eating regimen known as Dietary Ways to deal with Stop Hypertension (Run) are on the whole great beginning stages for a diabetic eating plan that can be changed to oblige your own eating inclinations.

These eating routine methodologies share two significant factors practically speaking: for the most part entire nourishments, and dinners worked around vegetables instead of sugars (carbs).

Be that as it may, as opposed to prevalent thinking—A diabetic eating routine isn't really a low-carb diet, nor should it be a high-protein or low-fat dinner plan. Indeed, ADA suggests less accentuation on explicit prerequisites for proteins, carbs, and fats, and more accentuation on following an entire nourishments approach that spotlights on the nature of your eating regimen; the less handled, refined, arranged, and quick nourishments centered, the better.

What's the serious deal about maintaining a strategic distance from handled nourishments? The more a nourishment has been precisely dealt with, and refined, the more noteworthy the probability that their dietary benefit will lower, and regularly has more sugar, refined flour, and immersed fats as their primary parts. By eating nourishments considered profoundly refined (ie, void calories), you are topping off on nourishments that will make it harder to deal with your weight and your glucose levels.

"A RD or CDE can take a gander at your standard eating routine and help you distinguish where there's opportunity to get better," Ms. Arevalo recommends. "These eating regimen specialists can likewise assist you with making a diabetes diet plan custom fitted to your own needs and nourishment inclinations."

At the point when you meet with a dietitian or CDE, she will consider the entirety of your wellbeing concerns, your weekday and end of the week plans, any social or strict inclinations, and your preferences, just as any other person who for the most part eats with you. By considering these variables, you will have the most obvious opportunity with regards to setting up a functional new way to deal with eating that will bolster your capacity to deal with your diabetes with the least interruption conceivable.

What You Have to Think About Eating with Diabetes

What amount do calories make a difference? For individuals with diabetes, the careful number of calories to expend every day depends on the sum and timing of nourishment that guarantees you can you're your glucose levels stable and your weight inside a sound range. That number can change, contingent upon your age, movement level, outline size, current versus favored weight, and different elements.

"At the point when the objective is a solid weight and glucose control, a great beginning stage for a lady is 1,400-1,600 calories every day, with principle dinners containing as much as 30 grams of fiber-rich sugars, and tidbits containing 10-20 grams of fiber-rich starches," Ms. Zanini prompts. "For men and all the more physically dynamic ladies who are as of now at a solid weight, you may begin with a 2,000-2,200 calorie feast plan, in which you may increment proportionately your carbs."

Ongoing exploration proposes that by having a major breakfast, and an unobtrusive lunch, so you get the greater part of your calories in by 3 pm, you will think that its simpler to get more fit and accomplish better glucose control.

Pick Starches that Keep Glucose Relentless

Our wide assortment of nourishment items contain various levels and sorts of sugars making it harder to eat astutely with diabetes. By and large, you will need to pick carbs that have minimal effect on your glucose. That implies choosing nourishments that are high fiber, low sugar nourishments since these nourishments are assimilated additionally easing back so have little effect on glucose changes.

Carbs and Their Effect on Diabetes

High fiber nourishments include: Entire grain breads and oats, and food sources made with 100% entire wheat, oats, quinoa, darker rice, corn and cornmeal, Dried beans, lentils, and peas

New (or solidified) organic products like berries, apples, pears, and oranges,

Dairy items including yogurt, milk, and cheddar. The best yogurt is Greek-style or stressed yogurt since these contain triple the degree of protein.

Vegetables: Both bland and non-dull vegetables are on the whole solid carbs that have less (glycemic) impact on your glucose

As you would figure, sugar-improved treats, cakes, doughnuts, and other prepared products made with white flour just as sweets and soda pops that contain sugar and high fructose corn syrup have minimal dietary benefit and are probably going to send your glucose taking off, so ought to eat them just every so often, if by any stretch of the imagination, and just in exceptionally modest quantities

The equivalent goes for yogurt. Better to dodge alleged organic product improved yogurts in light of the fact that these are for the most part included sugar. Rather mix in some new or solidified berries, banana, or your preferred regular natural product to plain yogurt; and you may even include some granola or hacked pecans for crunch and a touch of included protein and fiber.

Flour and sugar speak to two fixings well on the way to unleash devastation for individuals with diabetes since they ordinarily include pointless calories, and wind up prompting a lift in glucose and your weight; a one-two punch. While you don't need to maintain a strategic distance from flour and sugar out and out, you must be aware of when and how regularly you are eating nourishments flour-based, sugary nourishments. Skip nourishments made with universally handy white flour and keep away from sugary nourishments, sugar-improved beverages.

A Word on Sugar Substitutes: The present conviction is that individuals who need to follow a diabetes diet ought to maintain a strategic distance from included sugars of various types, including sugar substitutes and fake sugars. Scientists have discovered that individuals who devour nourishments with any type of sugar ordinarily pine for a greater amount of these nourishments, and wind up putting on weight.

Your most logical option is to start utilizing organic product to get your sweet fix. By adding natural product to nourishments, you thoroughly maintain a strategic distance from the additional sugars and sugar alcohols and get the additional advantage of dietary fiber, which is better for blood glucose control.

"Of all the elective sugars, stevia is the one I suggest regularly," says Ms. Zanini. "It's an extraordinary normal and zero-calorie choice for glucose control when added to refreshments, hot grains, and different nourishments when you are searching for a little sweetness." You'll need to try different things with stevia, she includes, in light of the fact that it works preferred with certain food sources over with others.

Probably the best change anybody with diabetes can change from white nourishment items—white bread, white potatoes in any structure, and white rice—which can likewise make outstanding spikes in glucose comparative items produced using entire grains, as multigrain sourdough bread, destroyed wheat or sweet potatoes, and broiled red potatoes which still have the skin on.

Figuring out how to set up your preferred hotcakes or waffles with oat flour or almond flour will go far in helping you to appreciate a diabetes-accommodating breakfast that the entire family will appreciate.

Carb Decisions Contain Dietary Fiber

This is the premise of a solid eating regimen, just as the way in to a diabetic eating routine arrangement, and even a decent eating routine for weight reduction. In the wake of perusing the area on carbs, it might be evident to you now that the one factor that isolates sound carbs from all different carbs is the nearness or nonappearance of dietary fiber. Just plant nourishments contain fiber. Those with the most fiber incorporate dried beans, peas, and lentils, organic products, vegetables, entire grains, nuts, and seeds.

A high fiber diet—one that contains in any event 25 to 35 grams of dietary fiber daily—is fundamental for acceptable wellbeing, and is the key for individuals with diabetes since fiber hinders the retention all things considered—those that are normally shaping like in products of the soil, just as any refined sugars you devour—in your circulation system.

"At the point when suppers are well-adjusted (counting some protein, fat and fiber-rich carbs), they are commonly additionally fulfilling," Ms. Zanini includes, which implies you won't get eager among suppers and go searching for a handy solution that will cause your glucose to take off, and your body to store those unneeded calories as fat.

Protein: Settle on Your Decisions Most reduced in Immersed Fat

Except if you are a veggie lover or vegetarian, you're probably going to get a lot of great protein from lean meats, poultry, fish, dairy, and eggs.

The two veggie lovers and non-vegans ought to likewise hope to plant hotspots for a few or the entirety of your protein needs. Plant nourishments like soy-based nourishments: tofu and tempeh are phenomenal wellsprings of non-creatures proteins and fits very well into a diabetic dinner plan since it is likewise low in carbs. The equivalent can be said for nuts, and vegetables, for example, dark beans, chickpeas, lentils, and edamame just as some entire grain nourishments, for example, quinoa, kamut, teff, even wild rice and couscous contain some protein.

Not All Fats Are Made Equivalent so Focus on Heart-Sound Fats

At the point when you have diabetes, you are at higher danger of creating other ceaseless medical issues, for example, coronary illness, hypertension, and kidney ailment, so it's similarly as imperative to watch the sorts and measures of fat in your eating routine all things considered to screen your carbs.

What nourishments contain heart-sound fats? These incorporate olive oil and oils produced using nuts (eg, pecan oil, nut oil), avocado, greasy fish l(eg, Sockeye salmon, mackerel, herring, and Lake trout), nuts and seeds.

Landing at Solid Eating routine that Meets Your Requirements with Diabetes

Since you recognize what nourishments are better in the event that you have diabetes, putting the correct nourishments on your plate involves parcels. The way in to a decent eating regimen is arranging suppers utilizing the diabetes plate technique—separate the plate into quarters: ¼ protein or meat, 1/4 carbs, and 2/4 (=1/2) vegetable and fruit.6 In the event that you need to get more fit, utilize 9-inch supper plates and bowls so you aren't heaping the nourishment on to a huge supper plate.

For instance, fill a large portion of the plate with non-bland carbs, for example, serving of mixed greens or steamed broccoli, and fill the staying half of the plate with equivalent bits of a grain or dull vegetable like pounded sweet potato, and a heart-sound protein, for example, cooked salmon.

Here are some example supper menus to give you a thought of sensible part evaluates that make a sound feast for somebody with diabetes (or anybody so far as that is concerned!):

Recommendation for Dinner:

- 5 or 6 ounces cooked chicken (skin expelled)

- 1/2 cup multigrain pasta (Cooked, or Bangz chickpea pasta) hurled with 2 tablespoons olive oil, and a teaspoon of ground Parmesan cheddar

- 2 cups sautéed zucchini as well as summer squash and cut mushrooms

- 6-ounce salmon filet, seared with lemon

- 1/2 cup daintily steamed broccoli and 1/2 cup split cherry tomatoes

- 1 cup child kale and spinach, daintily sautéed in olive oil with cleaved garlic and onion

- 6 ounces (around 1/2 cups) sauteed tofu prepared with Chinese 5-zest powder

- 1/3 cup quinoa

- 1/4 avocado, cut and beat with sesame seeds and a press of lime

- 1 cup cucumber, snow pea pods, arugula, and radish serving of mixed greens dressed with vinegar and light soy sauce

Step by step instructions to Respond When Enticement Hits with Diabetes

In diabetes diet terms, allurement means nourishments you "shouldn't" eat on the grounds that they are stacked with sugar and void carbs that will send your glucose soaring. That bit of cake, cinnamon bun, brownie, or sack of chips for the most part contain something other than carbs, they as a rule contribute undesirable fats as well.

The less frequently you eat these sugary, greasy sweets and tidbits, the less you will come to need them. A few people improve permitting yourself an incidental hankering. Finding some kind of harmony will rely on your objectives, and desperation. By skirting these calorie-loaded conduit cloggers, you are deciding in favor of long haul wellbeing instead of genuine restorative inconveniences. In any case, you realize that as of now.

Listen to this: this expression of alert isn't only for individuals with diabetes who need to watch their sugar and fat admission, in truth, it is a warning for any individual who needs remain solid and stay away from incessant ailments. That is the reason the entire family profits by eating well nourishments and sparing little guilty pleasures for exceptional events.

The most effective method to Partake in Festivities with Diabetes

Let's be honest, being encompassed by cupcakes and chips while others get their fill at birthday celebrations and special festivals, can be extremely disappointing. There are a few things you can do to overcome these occasions without feeling totally denied. In the first place, you can ensure you have been eating adjusted dinners before in the day, so you land at the occasion with a settled glucose, and not starving.

"You don't need to quit eating desserts so as to control your glucose and, truth be told, on the off chance that you include these "additional items" deliberately, you'll improve your odds of long haul achievement," Ms. Zanini says. "Giving yourself consent to appreciate an infrequent sweet may enable you to self-oversee diabetes such that suits your individual needs."

The way to eating with diabetes is to eat an assortment of solid nourishments from all nutrition types, in the sums your dinner plan plots.

The nutrition classes are

Vegetables

Non-starchy: incorporates broccoli, carrots, greens, peppers, and tomatoes

Boring: incorporates potatoes, corn, and green peas

Organic products—incorporates oranges, melon, berries, apples, bananas, and grapes

Grains—at any rate half of your grains for the day ought to be entire grains

Incorporates wheat, rice, oats, cornmeal, grain, and quinoa

Models: bread, pasta, oat, and tortillas

Protein

Lean meat

Chicken or turkey without the skin

Fish

Eggs

Nuts and peanuts

Dried beans and certain peas, for example, chickpeas and split peas

Meat substitutes, for example, tofu

Dairy—nonfat or low fat

Milk or sans lactose milk on the off chance that you have lactose narrow mindedness

Yogurt

Cheddar

Eat nourishments with heart-solid fats, which chiefly originate from these nourishments: Oils that are fluid at room temperature, for example, canola and olive oil , nuts and seeds, heart-solid fish, for example, salmon, fish, and mackerel, avocado

Use oils when preparing nourishment rather than spread, cream, shortening, grease, or stick margarine.

Pick sound fats, for example, from nuts, seeds, and olive oil.

Part estimates

You can utilize regular items or your hand to pass judgment on the size of a part.

- 1 serving of meat or poultry is the palm of your hand or a deck of cards

- 1 3-ounce serving of fish is a checkbook

- 1 serving of cheddar is six shakers

- 1/2 cup of cooked rice or pasta is an adjusted bunch or a tennis ball

- 1 serving of a flapjack or waffle is a DVD

- 2 tablespoons of nutty spread is a ping-pong ball

Some Meals and Supplements to Avoid as a Diabetes patient

Diabetes is a chronic disease that has reached epidemic proportions among adults and children worldwide. Uncontrolled diabetes has many serious consequences, including heart disease, kidney disease, blindness and other complications.

Prediabetes has also been linked to these conditions. Importantly, eating the wrong foods can raise your blood sugar and insulin levels and promote inflammation, which may increase your risk of disease.

A portion of the most noticeably terrible meals for diabetes – the food sources that raise glucose, decrease insulin affectability and increment type 2 diabetes chance – are the food sources that are generally regular in the standard American eating regimen.

Over time, high levels can damage your body's nerves and blood vessels, which may set the stage for heart disease, kidney disease and other serious health conditions.

Maintaining a low carb intake can help prevent blood sugar spikes and greatly reduce the risk of diabetes complications.

Therefore, it's important to avoid the foods listed below.

Sugar-Sweetened Beverages

Sugary beverages are the worst drink choice for someone with diabetes.

To begin with, they are very high in carbs, with a 12-ounce (354-ml) can of soda providing 38 grams .

The same amount of sweetened iced tea and lemonade each contain 36 grams of carbs, exclusively from sugar.

In addition, they're loaded with fructose, which is strongly linked to insulin resistance and diabetes. Indeed, studies suggest that consuming sugar-sweetened beverages may increase the risk of diabetes-related conditions like fatty liver.

What's more, the high fructose levels in sugary drinks may lead to metabolic changes that promote belly fat and potentially harmful cholesterol and triglyceride levels.

In one study of overweight and obese adults, consuming 25% of calories from high-fructose beverages on a weight-maintaining diet led to increased insulin resistance and belly fat, lower metabolic rate and worse heart health markers.

To help control blood sugar level and prevent disease risk, consume water, club soda or unsweetened iced tea instead of sugary beverages.

Diabetes is portrayed by strangely raised blood glucose levels. So it's shrewd to maintain a strategic distance from nourishments that cause hazardously high spikes in blood glucose. These are essentially refined nourishments, for example, sugar-improved refreshments, without fiber that eases back the ingestion of glucose in the blood.

Organic product juices and sugary prepared nourishments and treats have comparable impacts. These nourishments advance hyperglycemia and insulin obstruction. Also, they advance the arrangement of cutting edge glycation final results (AGEs) in the body.

AGEs adjust the ordinary, sound capacity of cell proteins, harden the veins, quicken maturing, and advance diabetes entanglements.

SUMMARY:

Sodas and sweet drinks are high in carbs, which increase blood sugar. Also, their high fructose content has been linked to insulin resistance and an increased risk of obesity, fatty liver and other diseases.

Trans Fats

Industrial trans fats are extremely unhealthy. They are created by adding hydrogen to unsaturated fatty acids in order to make them more stable.

Trans fats are found in margarines, peanut butter, spreads, creamers and frozen dinners. In addition, food manufacturers often add them to crackers, muffins and other baked goods to help extend shelf life.

Although trans fats don't directly raise blood sugar levels, they've been linked to increased inflammation, insulin resistance and belly fat, as well as lower "good" HDL cholesterol levels and impaired arterial function. These effects are especially concerning for people with diabetes, as they are at an increased risk of heart disease.

Fortunately, trans fats have been outlawed in most countries, and in 2015 the FDA called for their removal from products in the US market to be completed within three years.

Until trans fats are no longer in the food supply, avoid any product that contains the words "partially hydrogenated" in its ingredient list.

Diabetes quickens cardiovascular sickness. Since most by far of diabetics (over 80%) kick the bucket from cardiovascular malady, any nourishment that builds cardiovascular hazard will be particularly tricky for those with diabetes.

Trans fat admission is a solid dietary hazard factor for coronary illness; even a modest quantity of trans fat admission expands chance.

Notwithstanding their cardiovascular impacts, immersed and trans fats lessen insulin affectability, prompting raised glucose and insulin levels, and more serious danger of diabetes.

SUMMARY:

Trans fats are unsaturated fats that have been chemically altered to increase their stability. They have been linked to inflammation, insulin resistance, increased belly fat and heart disease.

White Bread, Pasta and Rice

White bread, rice and pasta are high-carb, processed foods. Eating bread, bagels and other refined-flour foods has been shown to significantly increase blood sugar levels in people with type 1 and type 2 diabetes.

What's more, this reaction isn't elite to wheat items. In one examination, without gluten pastas were additionally appeared to raise glucose, with rice-based sorts having the best impact.

Another examination found that a supper containing a high-carb bagel raised glucose as well as diminished cerebrum work in individuals with type 2 diabetes and mental shortages. These handled nourishments contain little fiber, which hinders the assimilation of sugar into the circulation system.

In another investigation, supplanting white bread with high-fiber bread was appeared to altogether decrease glucose levels in individuals with diabetes. Likewise, they encountered decreases in cholesterol and circulatory strain.

SUMMARY:

White bread, pasta and rice are high in carbs yet low in fiber. This blend can bring about high glucose levels. Then again, picking high-fiber, entire nourishments may help lessen glucose reaction.

Natural product Enhanced Yogurt

Plain yogurt can be a decent alternative for individuals with diabetes. In any case, organic product enhanced assortments are an altogether different story.

Seasoned yogurts are ordinarily produced using non-fat or low-fat milk and stacked with carbs and sugar.

Indeed, a one-cup (245-gram) serving of organic product enhanced yogurt may contain 47 grams of sugar, which means almost 81% of its calories originate from sugar.

Numerous individuals believe solidified yogurt to be a sound choice to frozen yogurt. In any case, it can contain the same amount of or much more sugar than frozen yogurt.

As opposed to picking high-sugar yogurts that can spike your glucose and insulin, select plain, entire milk yogurt that contains no sugar and might be advantageous for your craving, weight control and gut wellbeing.

SUMMARY:

Natural product seasoned yogurts are normally low in fat however high in sugar, which can prompt higher glucose and insulin levels. Plain, entire milk yogurt is a superior decision for diabetes control and in general wellbeing.

Improved Breakfast Grains

Eating grain is one of the most exceedingly terrible approaches to begin your day on the off chance that you have diabetes.

In spite of the wellbeing claims on their crates, most grains are profoundly handled and contain definitely more carbs than numerous individuals figure it out.

What's more, they give almost no protein, a supplement that can assist you with feeling full and fulfilled while keeping your glucose levels stable during the day.

Indeed "sound" breakfast grains aren't acceptable decisions for those with diabetes.

For example, only a half-cup serving (55 grams) of granola grain contains 30 grams of absorbable carbs, and Grape Nuts contain 41 grams. Likewise, each gives just 7 grams of protein for every serving. To monitor glucose and appetite, avoid the oat and pick a protein-based low-carb breakfast.

SUMMARY:

Breakfast grains are high in carbs yet low in protein. A high-protein, low-carb breakfast is the best choice for diabetes and hunger control.

Seasoned Espresso Beverages

Espresso has been connected to a few medical advantages, including a diminished danger of diabetes. In any case, enhanced espresso beverages ought to be seen as a fluid sweet, as opposed to a solid drink.

Studies have demonstrated your cerebrum doesn't process fluid and strong nourishments comparatively. At the point when you drink calories, you don't repay by eating less later, possibly prompting weight increase.

Seasoned espresso drinks are likewise stacked with carbs. Indeed "light" variants contain enough carbs to altogether raise your glucose levels.

For example, a 16-ounce (454-ml) caramel frappuccino from Starbucks contains 67 grams of carbs, and a similar size caramel light frappuccino contains 30 grams of carbs.

To monitor your glucose and forestall weight gain, pick plain espresso or coffee with a tablespoon of overwhelming cream or creamer.

SUMMARY:

Seasoned espresso drinks are exceptionally high in fluid carbs, which can raise glucose levels and neglect to fulfill your yearning.

Red and Prepared Meats

From the start, it might appear as though the dietary impacts on diabetes would be just applicable to sugar containing nourishments. The more low-sugar, high-protein nourishments in your eating regimen, the better; those nourishments don't straightforwardly raise blood glucose.

Notwithstanding, that is a too shortsighted perspective on the improvement of type 2 diabetes. Type 2 diabetes isn't just determined by raised glucose levels, yet additionally by constant irritation, oxidative pressure, and modifications in coursing lipids (fats).

Numerous diabetics have come to accept that if sugar and refined grains and other high-glycemic nourishments raise glucose and triglycerides, they ought to stay away from them and eat progressively creature protein to hold their blood glucose levels under tight restraints.

Notwithstanding, a few examinations have now affirmed that high admission of meat expands the danger of diabetes.

A meta-examination of 12 investigations inferred that high complete meat consumption expanded sort 2 diabetes hazard 17% above low admission, high red meat admission expanded hazard 21%, and high handled meat admission expanded hazard 41%.

Nectar, Agave Nectar and Maple Syrup

Individuals with diabetes regularly attempt to limit their admission of white table sugar, just as treats like sweets, treats and pie.

Notwithstanding, different types of sugar can likewise cause glucose spikes. These incorporate dark colored sugar and "characteristic" sugars like nectar, agave nectar and maple syrup.

Despite the fact that these sugars aren't profoundly handled, they contain at any rate the same number of carbs as white sugar. Actually, most contain much more.

The following are the carb tallies of a one-tablespoon serving of famous sugars:

White sugar: 12.6 grams

Agave nectar: 16 grams

Nectar: 17 grams

Maple syrup: 13 grams

In one examination, individuals with prediabetes experienced comparative increments in glucose, insulin and fiery markers whether or not they devoured 1.7 ounces (50 grams) of white sugar or nectar.

Your best system is to stay away from all types of sugar and utilize normal low-carb sugars.

SUMMARY:

Nectar, agave nectar and maple syrup are not as prepared as white table sugar, however they may effectsly affect glucose, insulin and fiery markers.

Dried Natural product

Natural product is an incredible wellspring of a few significant nutrients and minerals, including nutrient C and potassium. At the point when natural product is dried, the procedure brings about lost water that prompts significantly higher convergences of these supplements.

Shockingly, its sugar content turns out to be progressively thought also.

One cup of grapes contains 27 grams of carbs, including 1 gram of fiber. On the other hand, one cup of raisins contains 115 grams of carbs, 5 of which originate from fiber.

In this manner, raisins contain multiple occasions the same number of carbs as grapes do. Different kinds of dried organic product are likewise higher in carbs when contrasted with crisp natural product.

In the event that you have diabetes, you don't need to surrender organic product by and large. Staying with low-sugar organic products like new berries or a little apple can give medical advantages while keeping your glucose in the objective range.

SUMMARY:

Dried natural products become increasingly amassed in sugar and may contain multiple occasions the same number of carbs as crisp organic products do. Maintain a strategic distance from dried products of the soil natural products low in sugar for ideal glucose control.

Bundled Nibble Nourishments

Pretzels, wafers and other bundled nourishments aren't acceptable nibble decisions.

They're normally made with refined flour and give not many supplements, in spite of the fact that they have a lot of quick processing carbs that can quickly raise glucose.

Here are the carb means a one-ounce (28-gram) serving of some well known bites:

Saltine wafers: 21 grams of carbs, including 1 gram of fiber

Pretzels: 22 grams of carbs, including 1 gram of fiber

Graham wafers: 21 grams of carbs, including 1 gram of fiber

Truth be told, a portion of these nourishments may contain much more carbs than expressed on their sustenance name. One examination found that nibble nourishments give 7.7% more carbs, by and large, than the name states.

On the off chance that you get eager in the middle of suppers, it's smarter to eat nuts or a couple of low-carb vegetables with an ounce of cheddar.

SUMMARY:

Bundled snacks are commonly exceptionally handled nourishments produced using refined flour that can rapidly raise your glucose levels.

Preventative Word on Salt

A few people are touchy to salt, which causes more severe hypertension when a lot of sodium is devoured. Since we have no chance to get of testing who is salt-touchy and who isn't, the best precautionary measure is to restrict salt and stay away from sodium-containing nourishments on the off chance that you might be in danger for hypertension.

Basically, the abundance salt in a great many people's eating regimens originates from handled nourishments so check the bundle for sodium content. By embracing a diabetes diet that contains for the most part entire nourishments, this issue will never again introduce an issue. Additionally, nourishments that are streak solidified are in the same class as new.

Canned vegetables for the most part have included salt as an additive. Your most logical option when purchasing nourishment items is to check the dietary mark for sodium content. You'll need to remain well underneath the upper suggested breaking point of 2,000 mg/day, and you can unquestionably search for low-sodium assortments of canned, and handled, prepackaged nourishment items.

Natural product Juice

In spite of the fact that organic product juice is frequently viewed as sound refreshment, its impacts on glucose are really like those of soft drinks and other sugary beverages. This goes for unsweetened 100% natural product juice, just as types that contain included sugar. At times, natural product juice is significantly higher in sugar and carbs than pop. For instance, 8 ounces (250 ml) of unsweetened squeezed apple and soft drink contain 24 grams of sugar each. A proportional serving of grape juice gives 32 grams of sugar.

Like sugar-improved drinks, organic product juice is stacked with fructose, the kind of sugar that drives insulin opposition, weight and coronary illness.

A vastly improved option is to appreciate water with a wedge of lemon, which gives under 1 gram of carbs and is for all intents and purposes without calorie.

SUMMARY:

Unsweetened organic product juice contains at any rate as a lot of sugar as soft drinks do. Its high fructose substance can decline insulin obstruction, advance weight addition and increment the danger of coronary illness.

Entire Eggs

Eating 5 eggs/week or more has been related with an expanded danger of creating type 2 diabetes.

With regards to coronary illness, eggs have been a dubious subject. Be that as it may, for those with diabetes, the examination isn't disputable; there are clear connections in numerous observational investigations to huge increments in hazard.

Huge imminent examinations, for example, The Medical attendants' Wellbeing Study, Wellbeing Experts Follow-up Study, and Doctors' Wellbeing Concentrate revealed that diabetics who eat more than one egg/day twofold their cardiovascular malady or demise hazard contrasted with diabetics that ate short of what one egg for each week.

Another investigation of diabetics revealed that those eating one egg/day or more had a fivefold increment in danger of death from cardiovascular sickness.

Refined Grains (White Rice and White Flour Items)

Sugars like white rice, white pasta, and white bread are feeling the loss of the fiber from the first grain. So they raise blood glucose higher and quicker than their flawless, natural partners.

In a six-year investigation of 65,000 ladies, those with slims down high in refined sugars from white bread, white rice, and pasta were 2.5 occasions as prone to be determined to have type 2 diabetes contrasted with the individuals who ate lower-glycemic-load nourishments, for example, unblemished entire grains and entire wheat bread.

An examination of four forthcoming investigations on white rice utilization and diabetes found that every day by day serving of white rice expanded the danger of diabetes by 11%.

Notwithstanding the glucose-raising impacts, cooked dull nourishments additionally contain AGEs, which advance maturing and diabetes entanglements.

Singed Nourishments

Potato chips, French fries, doughnuts, and other singed starches start with a high-glycemic nourishment, and afterward heap on countless low-supplement calories as oil.

Also, as other cooked starches, singed nourishments contain AGEs.

They are nourishments to avoid, particularly on the off chance that you have diabetes. Potatoes themselves are moderately high in carbs. One medium potato with the skin on contains 37 grams of carbs, 4 of which originate from fiber. Notwithstanding, when they've been stripped and singed in vegetable oil, potatoes may accomplish more than spike your glucose.

Profound fricasseeing nourishments has been appeared to deliver high measures of poisonous mixes like AGEs and aldehydes, which may advance irritation and increment the danger of ailment. To be sure, a few investigations have connected often devouring french fries and other seared nourishments to coronary illness and disease. In the event that you would prefer not to keep away from potatoes by and large, eating a modest quantity of sweet potatoes is your best alternative.

Make substitutions

Try not to agree to what accompanies your sandwich or feast.

Rather than french fries, pick a diabetes-accommodating side plate of mixed greens or a twofold request of a vegetable.

Utilize sans fat or low-fat plate of mixed greens dressing, as opposed to the customary assortment, or attempt a crush of lemon juice, enhanced vinegar or salsa on your serving of mixed greens.

Request salsa or pico de gallo — an uncooked salsa — with your burrito rather than destroyed cheddar and harsh cream.

On a sandwich, exchange house dressings or smooth sauces for ketchup, mustard, horseradish or new tomato cuts.

SUMMARY:

Notwithstanding being high in carbs that raise glucose levels, french fries are seared in undesirable oils that may advance aggravation and increment the danger of coronary illness and malignant growth.

Pure fats: Maintain a strategic distance from high-fat dairy items and creature proteins, for example, margarine, meat, franks, wiener and bacon. Likewise limit coconut and palm piece oils.

Cholesterol: Cholesterol sources incorporate high-fat dairy items and high-fat creature proteins, egg yolks, liver, and other organ meats. Focus on close to 200 milligrams (mg) of cholesterol daily.

Sodium: Focus on under 2,300 mg of sodium daily. Your PCP may propose you focus on even less on the off chance that you have hypertension.

The Main concern

Knowing which nourishments to keep away from when you have diabetes can some of the time appear to be intense. Be that as it may, following a couple of rules can make it simpler.

Your fundamental objectives ought to incorporate avoiding unfortunate fats, fluid sugars, prepared grains and different nourishments that contain refined carbs.

Maintaining a strategic distance from nourishments that expansion your glucose levels and drive insulin opposition can help keep you solid now and decrease your danger of future diabetes intricacies.

To find out about the best nourishments to eat on the off chance that you have diabetes, look at this article.

Conclusion

The way to fortifying eating just everything when it comes to managing individuals with diabetes, is to eat an assortment of refreshing nourishments from every one of the nutrition classes and to maintain a strategic distance from profoundly prepared meals that contain high sugar, salt, and fat.

Notwithstanding the sorts of nourishment in an individual's present eating routine, a lot of energizing choices are accessible to attempt. When an individual has changed in accordance with another eating routine, they may not miss the nourishments that they used to eat.

A diabetes instructor or dietitian can help with building up a refreshing eating plan. They can prescribe what nourishments to eat, the amount to eat, and when to have dinners and bites. They will put together these proposals with respect to different components, including weight, physical action level, drugs, and blood glucose targets.

Find the best eating routine for diabetics and how to eat to forestall diabetes. Type 2 diabetes can be turned around — and even sort 1 diabetics can improve their life and wellbeing.

Diabetes is the seventh driving reason for death in the U.S. also, pairs the danger of coronary episode and stroke. It negatively affects the strength of our populace. Also, it quickens maturing; harming the kidneys, cardiovascular framework, eyes and nerve tissue, and builds disease hazard.

In any case, type 2 diabetes is a way of life ailment — our nourishment decisions can either forestall or advance insulin obstruction and resultant diabetes.

Counteraction is conceivable with regards to the overwhelming entanglements and unexpected losses related with diabetes. The essential driver of the parallel increments in weight and diabetes is the supplement exhausted American eating regimen. For diabetics and prediabetics particularly, new research demonstrates what mothers having been telling their kids through the ages, "eat your veggies, they're beneficial for you."

Incredible Physical Activities People with Diabetics can Engage in to Stay Fit

On the off chance that you have diabetes, these wellness thoughts can assist you with battling fat, increment bulk, improve balance, and diminish pressure — and may even decrease your requirement for insulin.

Do you get enough exercise? In case you're similar to numerous Americans, the appropriate response is no — and that is particularly valid for those of us with diabetes. Studies appear as not many as 39 percent of individuals with type 2 diabetes take part in ordinary physical action, contrasted and 58 percent of different Americans. Exercise additionally causes you get thinner and improve balance, which is significant in light of the fact that numerous individuals with type 2 diabetes are in danger for stoutness and for falls. "I completely prescribe that anybody more than 40 with diabetes incorporate parity preparing as a major aspect of their week after week schedule, in any event a few days out of each week," says Dr. Colberg-Ochs. "It tends to be as basic as working on adjusting on each leg in turn, or progressively intricate — like judo works out. Lower body and center opposition practices likewise twofold as parity preparing."

Here are six extraordinary exercises you can without much of a stretch work into your every day schedule. Make certain to check with your primary care physician before starting any activity routine, and go gradually from the start. After some time, you can build the length and force of your daily schedule.

Swimming

Swimming is another vigorous exercise — and a perfect one for individuals with type 2 diabetes since it doesn't squeeze your joints. "Being floated by the water is less distressing for you," according to Colberg-Ochs. Swimming additionally is simpler on your feet than different types of activity, for example, strolling or running. Regularly diabetes lessens blood stream to the little veins of your furthest points and you can lose sensation in your feet thus. Individuals with diabetes must maintain a strategic distance from foot wounds, even minor cuts or rankles, in light of the fact that they can be delayed to mend and are inclined to disease. Exceptional shoes made for use in the pool can help forestall scratched feet and decrease the danger of slipping.

Martial Art

Kendo, a progression of developments acted in a moderate and loosened up way more than 30 minutes, has been polished for a considerable length of time. At any rate one little examination has affirmed it is an incredible decision of activity for type 2 diabetes. Kendo is perfect for individuals with diabetes since it gives wellness and stress decrease in one. Judo likewise improves balance and may decrease nerve harm, a typical diabetic difficulty — however the last advantage "stays dubious," says Colberg-Ochs. In any case, she accentuates that taking a shot at your parity every day is a basic part of remaining on your feet as you age, and living admirably and autonomously all through your lifetime. "On the off chance that you don't do judo, join some other parity practices into your week by week schedule to lessen your danger of falling," says Colberg-Ochs.

Light Weight lifting

"I can't say enough regarding the advantages of weight preparing, for individuals with diabetes as well as for everybody," Colberg-Ochs says. Weight preparing assembles bulk, significant for those with type 2 diabetes. "On the off chance that you lose bulk, you have significantly harder time keeping up your glucose," Colberg-Ochs says. Plan for obstruction exercise or weight preparing in any event two times per week as a major aspect of your diabetic administration plan — three is perfect, yet consistently plan a rest day between weight exercises (other exercise is fine on those days). Every session ought to incorporate 5 to 10 distinct sorts of lifting including the significant muscle gatherings. For ideal quality additions, stir your way up to doing three to four arrangements of each activity, with each set containing 10 to 15 redundancies.

Strolling

Strolling is simple for individuals to do, All you need is a decent pair of shoes and some place to go. Strolling is likely one of the most recommended exercises for individuals with type 2 diabetes. Energetic strolling done at a pace that raises the pulse is an oxygen consuming activity, and studies show gainful impacts when individuals with diabetes take an interest in high-impact exercises in any event three days per week for an aggregate of 150 minutes. The American Diabetes Affiliation (ADA) suggests individuals not go in excess of two continuous days without an oxygen consuming activity session.

Yoga

Various examinations show that on the off chance that you have diabetes, yoga can profit you in a few different ways. It can assist lower with bodying fat, battle insulin obstruction, and improve nerve work — immeasurably significant when you have type 2 diabetes. Like judo, yoga is additionally an extraordinary diabetic pressure reducer. "At the point when feelings of anxiety go higher, so do your glucose levels," says Colberg-Ochs.

One of the benefits of yoga as an activity is that you can do it as regularly as you like. "The more the better," she says. An investigation distributed in Walk 2017 in the Diary of Physical Movement and Wellbeing finished up practice decreases burdensome indications in grown-ups with type 2 diabetes, and proposed that less exercise might be required for individuals who are stout so as to accomplish significant outcomes.

Tips to Stay Safe while Exercising

Continuously counsel with your primary care physician before starting any activity program to be certain it is medicinally protected to exercise and audit standards noted underneath.

Exercise can bring down glucose out of nowhere, yet on account of solidarity preparing, it can expand glucose levels. Make certain to screen glucose levels when all activity schedules to all the more likely see how your body reacts to practice and to forestall any serious deviations.

Those with Type 1 diabetes ought to likewise test for ketones in their pee (if glucose is harshly or unexplainably high) before practicing and ought to keep away from incredible movement/practice when ketones are raised. You can almost certainly practice when your glucose is high as long as there are no ketones in your pee and glucose isn't seriously high.

For those taking insulin and additionally drugs, for example, glipizide or glyburide (insulin secretagogues), exercise can cause low glucose if prescription portion or starch admission isn't balanced suitably. Additional starches should probably be devoured if pre-practice glucose levels are under 100 to 120 mg/dL.

Low glucose is less regular in diabetic patients who are not treated with insulin or insulin secretagogues, and no preventive measures for low glucose are normally required in these cases.

When you feel any of these symptoms while exercising, it is very important to stop and seek for medical assistance.

- Serious or unordinary weariness or sluggishness
- Tipsiness or wooziness
- Restlessness
- Bizarre brevity of breath
- Fast heart beat
- Chest distress
- Jaw, arm, or upper back distress
- Serious distress of any sort

The Most ideal Approach to manage Diabetes and Upgrade Future

Figuring out how to eat to forestall diabetes and how to eat on the off chance that you have diabetes or prediabetes can assist you with assuming responsibility for your wellbeing.

An eating regimen of vegetables, nuts, seeds, beans, and crisp natural product can forestall and even turn around diabetes while advancing long haul wellbeing. This methodology works. In an ongoing report on type 2 diabetics following this eating routine, we found that 90% of members had the option to fall off every diabetic prescription, and the mean HbA1c following one year was 5.8, which is in the non-diabetic (typical) go.

Become familiar with utilizing these nourishments to battle diabetes in my book The Finish of Diabetes. In this book, I layout my arrangement for forestalling and turning around type 2 diabetes utilizing prevalent nourishment, not drugs.

Nobody must have type 2 diabetes, and those with type 1 diabetes can improve their future, wellbeing and personal satisfaction with this arrangement.

In the event that you are aware of anybody with diabetes – type 1, type 2 or prediabetes – it is significant they perused this book; it could spare their life.

Nourishment can regularly be readied utilizing more beneficial strategies. Rather than having something breaded and singed, inquire as to whether your nourishment can be:

- Cooked
- Simmered
- Barbecued
- Steamed

- Different substitutions you should inquire as to whether the culinary expert can utilize include:
- Entire grain bread or pasta rather than white assortments
- Dark colored rice rather than white rice
- Skinless chicken
- Less oil, margarine or cheddar
- Veggies on a slight covering pizza

You don't have to feel unsure about mentioning more beneficial alternatives or substitutions. You're taking the necessary steps to remain focused on your treatment objectives. Furthermore, most cafés need to satisfy clients.

Spare space for dessert

Pastry isn't really beyond reach since you have diabetes. Natural product can be a decent decision, however on the off chance that you'd like a sweet other than organic product, make it part of your feast design and remunerate by lessening the measure of different sugars —, for example, bread, tortillas, rice, milk or potatoes — in your dinner. Or on the other hand think about offering a treat to somebody.

Starch tallying

Starch tallying includes monitoring the measure of sugars you eat and drink every day. Since starches transform into glucose in your body, they influence your blood glucose level more than different nourishments do. Carb tallying can assist you with dealing with your blood glucose level. In the event that you take insulin, tallying starches can assist you with realizing how much insulin to take.

The perfect measure of sugars changes by how you deal with your diabetes, including how physically dynamic you are and what medications you take, assuming any. Your social insurance group can assist you with making an individual eating plan dependent on starch tallying.

The measure of starches in nourishments is estimated in grams. To include starch grams in what you eat, you'll have to realize which nourishments have sugars peruse the Sustenance Certainties nourishment mark, or figure out how to appraise the quantity of grams of sugar in the nourishments you eat include the grams of sugar from every nourishment you eat to get your aggregate for every dinner and for the afternoon.

Most sugars originate from starches, organic products, milk, and desserts. Attempt to confine starches with included sugars or those with refined grains, for example, white bread and white rice. Rather, eat starches from natural product, vegetables, entire grains, beans, and low-fat or nonfat milk.

Pick solid sugars, for example, organic product, vegetables, entire grains, beans, and low-fat milk, as a major aspect of your diabetes supper plan. Notwithstanding utilizing the plate strategy and carb tallying, you might need to visit an enlisted dietitian (RD) for therapeutic sustenance treatment.

Plan ahead

Converse with your medicinal services group before you start another physical action schedule, particularly in the event that you have other medical issues. Your human services group will disclose to you an objective range for your blood glucose level and recommend how you can be dynamic securely.

Your human services group additionally can assist you with choosing the best time of day for you to do physical action dependent on your day by day plan, supper plan, and diabetes prescriptions. In the event that you take insulin, you have to adjust the movement that you do with your insulin dosages and dinners so you don't get low blood glucose.

Prevent low blood glucose

Because physical activity lowers your blood glucose, you should protect yourself against low blood glucose levels, also called hypoglycemia. You are most likely to have hypoglycemia if you take insulin or certain other diabetes medicines, such as a sulfonylurea. Hypoglycemia also can occur after a long intense workout or if you have skipped a meal before being active. Hypoglycemia can happen during or up to 24 hours after physical activity.

Planning is key to preventing hypoglycemia. For instance, if you take insulin, your health care provider might suggest you take less insulin or eat a small snack with carbohydrates before, during, or after physical activity, especially intense activity. You may need to check your blood glucose level before, during, and right after you are physically active.

Stay safe when blood glucose is high

If you have type 1 diabetes, avoid vigorous physical activity when you have ketones in your blood or urine. Ketones are chemicals your body might make when your blood glucose level is too high, a condition called hyperglycemia, and your insulin level is too low. If you are physically active when you have ketones in your blood or urine, your blood glucose level may go even higher. Ask your health care team what level of ketones are dangerous for you and how to test for them. Ketones are uncommon in people with type 2 diabetes.

Take care of your feet

People with diabetes may have problems with their feet because of poor blood flow and nerve damage that can result from high blood glucose levels. To help prevent foot problems, you should wear comfortable, supportive shoes and take care of your feet before, during, and after physical activity.

Add extra activity to your daily routine

If you have been inactive or you are trying a new activity, start slowly, with 5 to 10 minutes a day. Then add a little more time each week. Increase daily activity by spending less time in front of a TV or other screen. Try these simple ways to add physical activities in your life each

Walk around while you talk on the phone or during TV commercials.

Do chores, such as work in the garden, rake leaves, clean the house, or wash the car.

Park at the far end of the shopping center parking lot and walk to the store.

Take the stairs instead of the elevator.

Make your family outings active, such as a family bike ride or a walk in a park.

If you are sitting for a long time, such as working at a desk or watching TV, do some light activity for 3 minutes or more every half hour.5 Light activities include

- Leg lifts or extensions
- Overhead arm stretches
- Desk chair swivels

- Torso twists
- Side lunges
- Walking in place

Weight Reduction Arranging

On the off chance that you are overweight or have corpulence, work with your medicinal services group to make a weight reduction plan. The Body Weight Organizer can assist you with fitting your calorie and physical action intends to reach and keep up your objective weight.

To get fit, you have to eat less calories and supplant less solid nourishments with nourishments lower in calories, fat, and sugar.

On the off chance that you have diabetes, are overweight or fat, and are intending to have an infant, you should attempt to lose any overabundance weight before you become pregnant. Become familiar with making arrangements for pregnancy in the event that you have diabetes.

Supper Plan techniques

Two regular approaches to assist you with arranging the amount to eat in the event that you have diabetes are the plate technique and sugar tallying, likewise called carb checking. Check with your medicinal services group about the strategy that is best for you.

Plate Technique

The plate technique causes you control your part estimates. You don't have to check calories. The plate technique shows the measure of every nutritional category you ought to eat. This technique works best for lunch and supper.

Utilize a 9-inch plate. Put non-starchy vegetables on half of the plate; a meat or other protein on one-fourth of the plate; and a grain or other starch on the last one-fourth. Starches incorporate dull vegetables, for example, corn and peas. You additionally may eat a little bowl of organic product or a bit of natural product, and drink a little glass of milk as remembered for your feast plan.

Photograph of a plate with cucumber and spinach on half of the plate, darker rice on one fourth of the plate, and prepared chicken on the last quarter. The plate technique shows the measure of every nutrition class you ought to eat.

You can discover a wide range of mixes of nourishment and more insights regarding utilizing the plate strategy from the American Diabetes Affiliation's Make Your Plate Outside connection. Your day by day eating plan additionally may incorporate little snacks between suppers.

Do aerobic exercise

Aerobic exercise is activity that makes your heart beat faster and makes you breathe harder. You should aim for doing aerobic exercise for 30 minutes a day most days of the week. You do not have to do all the activity at one time. You can split up these minutes into a few times throughout the day.

To get the most out of your activity, exercise at a moderate to vigorous level. Try

- Walking briskly or hiking
- Climbing stairs
- Swimming or a water-aerobics class
- Dancing
- Riding a bicycle or a stationary bicycle

- Taking an exercise class
- Playing basketball, tennis, or other sports
- Talk with your health care team about how to warm up and cool down before and after you exercise.

Do strength training to build muscle

Strength training is a light or moderate physical activity that builds muscle and helps keep your bones healthy. Strength training is important for both men and women. When you have more muscle and less body fat, you'll burn more calories. Burning more calories can help you lose and keep off extra weight.

You can do strength training with hand weights, elastic bands, or weight machines. Try to do strength training two to three times a week. Start with a light weight. Slowly increase the size of your weights as your muscles become stronger.

You can do strength training with hand weights, elastic bands, or weight machines.

Do stretching exercises

Stretching exercises are light or moderate physical activity. When you stretch, you increase your flexibility, lower your stress, and help prevent sore muscles.

You can choose from many types of stretching exercises. Yoga is a type of stretching that focuses on your breathing and helps you relax. Even if you have problems moving or balancing, certain types of yoga can help. For instance, chair yoga has stretches you can do when sitting in a chair or holding onto a chair while standing. Your health care team can suggest whether yoga is right for you.

Learn the keys to healthy eating.

Knowing what to eat can be confusing. Everywhere you turn, there is news about what is or isn't good for you. But a few basic tips have withstood the test of time. Regardless of what cuisine you prefer, here's what all healthy eating plans have in common. They include:

- Fruits and vegetables
- Lean meats and plant-based sources of protein
- Less added sugar
- Less processed foods

Diabetes Meals to Try at A Resturant

Eating out is fun and advantageous, however in the event that you have diabetes, adhering to your sustenance plan while eating out can be a test. Luckily, numerous eateries presently offer sound decisions. In addition, menus and nourishment data are regularly accessible internet, enabling you to arrange for what you need before you even find a workable pace.

Regardless of whether you're eating at home or eating out, follow the nourishment rules built up by your primary care physician or enlisted dietitian, for example,

- Eat an assortment of sound nourishments, for example, vegetables and products of the soil fiber food sources
- Point of confinement the measure of unfortunate fat in your eating regimen, particularly trans fats
- Point of confinement the measure of salt you eat
- Keep desserts, for example, prepared products, sweet and frozen yogurt, to a base
- Development helps, as well.

Truly, you can eat out—basically anyplace! Here's the means by which to settle on keen decisions.

At the point when you have diabetes, eating out can appear to be more muddled than unraveling the new duty code. Be that as it may, it doesn't need to be.

"Individuals with diabetes can appreciate most any sort of eatery," says Jill Weisenberger, RDN, CDE, creator of Diabetes Weight reduction step by step. "The key is to adhere as near your typical supper plan as could reasonably be expected." Here's the ticket.

Check the café's site to check whether the menu and nourishment data are accessible on the web. These are acceptable instruments to get ready what you'll arrange. On the off chance that this data isn't on the web, take a stab at calling the eatery to inquire as to whether nourishments can be made with less salt, fat or sugar.

Pizza

Stressed over such outside? Go with one cut of flimsy covering pizza and you'll help the carb tally of your cut by a third contrasted with a customary cut. On the off chance that a solitary cut sounds excessively scanty, siphon up the volume—and the fiber—by including a lot of cleaved veggies. Furthermore, talking about veggies, topping off on a plate of mixed greens before your pie shows up can likewise place the breaks on hunger.

These pita pizzas will absolutely change the manner in which you consider supper:

"Given that pasta is pressed with sugars, it's most likely not the best plan to make it the focal point of your feast," says Weisenberger. Only one request for spaghetti and meatballs can undoubtedly pack 150 grams of carbs.

That doesn't mean you need to go 100% without pasta however. Weisenberger suggests requesting pasta as a side dish and constraining your part to a half-cup, or about the size of a tennis ball. Pair it with a request for mussels fra diavolo, chicken cacciatore, or flame broiled calamari. (What's more, ensure you attempt these 6 different ways to make Italian nourishment level stomach neighborly!)

Chinese

In case you're eating Chinese nourishment, odds are there will be rice on your plate. Also, if that rice is white, be set up for a significant glucose spike. White rice is irksome to such an extent that one investigation found that for each serving an individual ate for every day, their danger of creating type 2 diabetes bounced by 11%.

Since Chinese nourishment simply isn't, well, Chinese nourishment without rice, go with a half-cup of the dark colored assortment. It's a decent wellspring of magnesium, a mineral that enables your body to utilize insulin all the more proficiently. Concerning the remainder of your plate, Weisenberger suggests beginning your dinner with either hot and acrid soup or steamed dumplings, and tailing it with a fundamental dish of moo goo gai container or steamed fish and veggies.

Japanese

Sushi may appear as though it's reasonable game, however recollect: It's enveloped by rice. Dark colored rice sushi can be a superior wagered, however regardless you'll need to watch its carb check. The best way to know without a doubt is to pick a café that makes their nourishment details accessible. On the off chance that that is impractical, stay with a smallish request of six pieces or, even better, choose a request for without carb sashimi with a side of edamame for a sound portion of glucose leveling protein.

Mexican

You know those monster tortillas Mexican eateries use to wrap your burrito? Every one packs a humongous 50 grams of carbs. What's more, that is not in any event, tallying the extra 40 grams you'll get from a powerful filling of rice. Why not skirt the tortilla and rice completely and attempt a bean-rich burrito bowl? Beans gloat a low glycemic record, which means they're gradually processed so they won't cause your glucose to soar. They're so glucose benevolent that one ongoing examination discovered individuals who ate some beans a day for a quarter of a year decreased their A1C (a proportion of long haul glucose control).

On the off chance that burrito bowls aren't your thing, attempt barbecued fish tacos or chicken fajitas, and request 6-inch corn tortillas. They have 28% less carbs than flour tortillas.

Steak

On the off chance that you have diabetes, your primary care physician has presumably as of now guided you to avoid soaked fat-substantial nourishments like steak, burgers, and sheep hacks. That is on the grounds that individuals with type 2 diabetes are up to multiple times bound to kick the bucket of coronary illness than those with ordinary glucose. Yet, there are still a lot of sound—and delectable—alternatives on steakhouse menus like shrimp mixed drink, broil chicken, barbecued salmon, or even lobster (simply chill out on the drawn margarine!). Request any of these in addition to a serving of mixed greens alongside a side of asparagus, broccoli, or Brussels grows.

Greek

At the point when you're watching your glucose, Greek nourishment can offer the best—or the most noticeably awful—of feasting out. Approval to lean, low-carb chicken souvlaki, Greek serving of mixed greens, giandes (a yummy Greek-style rendition of prepared beans), and avegolemono (a.k.a. chicken orzo soup). Also, maintain a strategic distance from those greasy top picks like gyros, moussaka, spanakopita, and singed calamari.

Indian

From sleek singed samosas to rice-based dishes, Indian nourishment can appear to be a significant minefield. Your technique: Burden up on lean protein. Lentil soup (these vegetables are ideal for keeping glucose consistent), dal (lentil stew), and chana masala (fiery chickpeas) are for the most part victors. In case you're longing for something meatier, pick the roasted chicken. It's marinated in a light, zesty yogurt sauce and afterward barbecued. What could be more advantageous than that?

Cafés will in general serve enormous segments, perhaps twofold what you ordinarily eat or more. Attempt to eat a similar size bits you would on the off chance that you were eating at home by:

- Picking the littlest feast size if the café offers choices: for instance, a lunch-sized dish
- Imparting dinners to an eating accomplice or two
- Mentioning a bring home compartment
- Making a dinner out of a serving of mixed greens or soup and a hors d'oeuvre
- Eating gradually with the goal that you'll feel full before you've eaten excessively

In case that is no joke "everything you can eat" buffet, it tends to be hard to oppose gorging. Indeed, even a modest quantity of numerous nourishments can signify heaps of calories. At the point when you're at a smorgasbord, the "plate" technique can help. Top off a large portion of your plate with nonstarchy vegetables, a quarter with a protein and the last quarter with a starch.

Additional Options include

Bacon bits, bread garnishes, cheeses and other additional items can attack diabetes sustenance objectives by rapidly expanding a dinner's calories and starches.

In case you're eating some place that offers free bread or tortilla chips on the table and they simply don't fit into your supper plan, ask the server not to bring them.

Beverages matter, as well

Sugar-improved pop, juice or milkshakes can add heaps of calories to your supper, particularly if the eatery offers free tops off. Rather than unhealthy beverages, great beverage alternatives include:

- Water
- Unsweetened frosted tea
- Unsweetened tea or espresso
- Shining water
- Mineral water
- Diet pop
- It's a smart thought to drink a glass of water before you eat to cause you to feel full sooner.
- Liquor and diabetes

In the event that your diabetes is all around oversaw and your primary care physician concurs, a periodic mixed beverage with a supper is normally fine. In any case, remember that liquor includes void calories.

In the event that you use insulin or different drugs that lower glucose, liquor can cause a possibly hazardous low glucose level. In the event that you utilize these drugs and drink liquor, make certain to eat something while at the same time drinking.

In the event that you drink liquor, pick choices with less calories and starches, for example,

- Light lager

- Dry wines
- Blended beverages made with without sugar blenders, for example, diet pop, diet tonic, club pop or seltzer

Farthest point your liquor to one beverage daily for ladies everything being equal and men more established than age 65, and up to two beverages per day for men age 65 and more youthful.

Eating simultaneously consistently can assist you with keeping up relentless glucose levels — particularly on the off chance that you take diabetes pills or insulin shots. In case you're eating out with others, follow these tips:

Request to plan the social affair at your typical supper time.

To abstain from hanging tight for a table, reserve a spot or attempt to maintain a strategic distance from times when the café is busiest.

On the off chance that you can't abstain from eating later than expected, make certain to have a tidbit available on the off chance that you create side effects of low glucose.

Frequent Questions and answers

Question: For what reason do you have to build up a smart dieting plan?

Answer: In the event that you have diabetes or prediabetes, your primary care physician will probably prescribe that you see a dietitian to assist you with building up a good dieting arrangement. The arrangement causes you control your (glucose), deal with your weight and control coronary illness hazard factors, for example, hypertension and high blood fats.

At the point when you eat additional calories and fat, your body makes an unwanted ascent in blood glucose. In the event that blood glucose isn't held within proper limits, it can prompt major issues, for example, a high blood glucose level (hyperglycemia) that, if constant, may prompt long haul complexities, for example, nerve, kidney and heart harm.

You can help keep your blood glucose level in a sheltered range by settling on sound nourishment decisions and following your dietary patterns.

For a great many people with type 2 diabetes, weight reduction likewise can make it simpler to control blood glucose and offers a large group of other medical advantages. On the off chance that you have to get more fit, a diabetes diet gives an efficient, nutritious approach to arrive at your objective securely.

Diabetes diet: Make your good dieting arrangement

Your diabetes diet is essentially a smart dieting plan that will assist you with controlling your glucose. Here's assistance beginning, from dinner wanting to checking sugars.

A diabetes diet just methods eating the most beneficial nourishments in moderate sums and adhering to normal eating times.

A diabetes diet is a good dieting arrangement that is normally wealthy in supplements and low in fat and calories. Key components are organic products, vegetables and entire grains. Actually, a diabetes diet is the best eating arrangement for most everybody.

Question: How might I settle on more advantageous decisions when eating out?

Answer: It tends to be trying to eat out, both due to the questions about what precisely a supper will contain as far as carbs and calories, yet in addition since eating out with companions or family can frequently prompt accidental strain to eat nourishments you would be in an ideal situation without, for example, dessert!

When eating out don't feel modest posing inquiries about what a dish contains or how it is readied.

Take a gander at menus online before you go.

Converse with your loved ones previously about your explanations behind practicing good eating habits. Reveal to them it's essential to your long haul wellbeing that you remain on your smart dieting design and ask them not to urge you to eat things that aren't beneficial for you. Loved ones are frequently simply attempting to show their adoration by needing you to appreciate a pastry, anyway mixed up that is. Assist them with understanding they can best assistance you by not making it increasingly hard to remain on track and by supporting you in your endeavors to take great consideration of yourself.

Offer a solitary pastry with the entire table and limit yourself to two nibbles.

Pick ethnic eateries, for example, Thai, sushi, or Indian foods with loads of vegetables and less refined sugars like pasta and bread; Then streamlining your segment of rice to 1 cup.

Question: What are the intricacies of type 2 diabetes?

Answer: Type 2 diabetes can prompt various entanglements, for example, kidney, nerve, and eye harm, just as coronary illness. It additionally implies cells are not accepting the glucose they requirement for solid working. An estimation called a HOMA Score (Homeostatic Model Evaluation) can tell specialists the general extent of these variables for a person with type 2 diabetes. Great glycemic control (that is, keeping sugar/starch admission low so glucose isn't high) can forestall long haul inconveniences of type 2 diabetes. An eating routine for individuals with type 2 diabetes additionally is alluded to as a diabetic eating regimen for type 2 diabetes and restorative nourishment treatment (MNT) for individuals with diabetes.

Question: Would I be able to drink alcohol in the event that I have type 2 diabetes?

Answer: For the vast majority with type 2 diabetes, the general rule for moderate liquor utilization applies. Research shows that one beverage for each day for ladies and two every day for men diminishes cardiovascular hazard and doesn't negatively affect diabetes. Nonetheless, alcohol can bring down glucose, and individuals with type 2 diabetes who are inclined to hypoglycemia, (For instance, those using insulin) ought to know about postponed hypoglycemia.

Approach to prevent hypoglycemia

Eat nourishment with mixed beverages to help limit the hazard: Blended beverages and mixed drinks frequently are made with sugars or squeezes, and contain a lot of starches so they will expand glucose levels. Wear a diabetes ready arm ornament with the goal that individuals know to offer nourishment on the off chance that you show hypoglycemic manifestations. It likewise is critical to realize that hypoglycemia manifestations regularly emulate those of inebriation.

Question: What does a diabetes diet include?

Answer: A diabetes diet depends on eating three dinners per day at customary occasions. This encourages you better utilize the insulin that your body delivers or gets past a drug.

An enrolled dietitian can assist you with assembling an eating regimen dependent on your wellbeing objectives, tastes and way of life. The person in question can likewise chat with you about how to improve your dietary patterns, for example, picking segment measures that suit the requirements for your size and action level.

Question: What Is a Decent Eating regimen for Type 2 Diabetes?

Answer: Indeed, a brilliant diabetes diet looks a ton like the good dieting arrangement specialists suggest for everybody: It incorporates eating bunches of fiber-rich foods grown from the ground, getting a charge out of entire grain starches with some restraint, powering up with fit protein, and eating a moderate measure of sound fats. What it comes down to is that "There is no 'diabetic eating regimen'," says Erin Palinski-

Swim, RD, CDE, creator of multi Day Diabetes Diet and Paunch Fat Eating routine For Fakers, and situated in Vernon, New Jersey. "The rules are fundamentally the equivalent for good dieting for everybody, with or without diabetes," she says.

All things considered, eating when you have diabetes requires making a few strides that are explicit to the ailment. Despite the fact that there is certainly not a one-size-fits-all eating arrangement, realizing the essentials is key for keeping up a high caliber of life, lessening the danger of entanglements, and possibly in any event, turning around diabetes.

Question: What would it be a good idea for you to Eat On the off chance that You Have Diabetes?

Answer: In truth, an eating regimen planned for lessening the dangers of diabetes is actually simply a healthfully adjusted feast plan planned for supporting keeping up glucose levels inside range and supporting a solid weight.

For those with prediabetes or type 2 diabetes, the principle focal point of a diabetes-centered eating regimen is being mindful to your weight. That stated, a diabetic eating routine is basically an eating approach that attempts to keep you solid, as isn't held uniquely for individuals with diabetes. Your entire family can appreciate similar dinners and bites, whether or not others have diabetes or not.

Indeed—There are a couple of nourishment choices that will matter more on the off chance that you do have diabetes. We furnish you with some broad rules to assist you with seeing how much and how regularly to eat so as to keep up relentless glucose levels. What's more, these proposals remain constant for any individual who has diabetes: type 1 diabetes and type 2 diabetes, just as prediabetes and gestational diabetes.

Diet truly does make a difference, a great deal!

Truth be told, on the off chance that you were as of late determined to have prediabetes or type 2 diabetes, by diminishing your weight by about 10%, you may even switch your diabetes, placing it into remission.

Question: What are the consequences of a diabetes diet?

Answer: Grasping your smart dieting plan is the most ideal approach to monitor your blood glucose level and forestall diabetes entanglements. What's more, on the off chance that you have to get thinner, you can tailor it to your particular objectives.

Beside dealing with your diabetes, a diabetes diet offers different advantages, as well. Since a diabetes diet prescribes liberal measures of natural products, vegetables and fiber, tailing it is probably going to diminish your danger of cardiovascular maladies and specific sorts of disease. What's more, devouring low-fat dairy items can lessen your danger of low bone mass later on.

On the off chance that you have diabetes, it's significant that you collaborate with your primary care physician and dietitian to make an eating plan that works for you. Utilize sound nourishments, divide control and booking to deal with your blood glucose level. On the off chance that you stray from your recommended diet, you risk fluctuating glucose levels and that's just the beginning genuine confusions.

Question: Why You Ought to Remember Fiber for Your Diabetes Supper Plan?

Answer: An astounding method to trim your waistline and settle glucose is going after nourishments high in fiber. Fiber isn't processed by the human body, so fiber-rich nourishments with starches don't raise glucose levels as fast since they are prepared all the more gradually. Fiber-rich nourishments can likewise assist you with feeling more full for more, supporting weight reduction, forestalling corpulence, and possibly averting conditions, for example, coronary illness and colon malignancy.

Shockingly, most grown-ups don't eat enough fiber. Regardless of whether an individual has diabetes or not, they should mean to follow similar proposals. Ladies ought to get at any rate 25 g of fiber for every day, while men need in any event 38 g for every day, Palinski-Swim says.

Question: What Are the Best Wellsprings of Sugars for Individuals With Type 2 Diabetes?

Answer: You can discover starches in entire grains, natural products, vegetables, vegetables and beans, and dairy. Try not to avoid them, either, as they supply essential nutrients, minerals, and fiber, the NIH calls attention to. Great wellsprings of carbs include:

Entire grains, similar to entire wheat pasta and bread, dark colored rice, cereal, and quinoa

Nonstarchy veggies, similar to peppers, eggplant, onion, and asparagus

Boring veggies are alright to eat with some restraint, simply mind the sugar content. Models incorporate sweet potatoes and corn.

Nonfat or low-fat dairy, as unsweetened yogurt and curds

Beans and vegetables, similar to dark beans, chickpeas, and lentils

Question: Why Does Carb Intake Matter for People With Diabetes?

Diabetes builds your danger of coronary illness and stroke by quickening the improvement of obstructed and solidified supply routes. Nourishments containing the accompanying can neutralize your objective of a heart-solid eating routine.

Carbs, protein and fat are the macronutrients that provide your body with energy. Of these three, carbs have the greatest effect on your blood sugar by far. This is because they are broken down into sugar, or glucose, and absorbed into your bloodstream.

Carbs include starches, sugar and fiber. However, fiber isn't digested and absorbed by your body in the same way other carbs are, so it doesn't raise your blood sugar.

Subtracting fiber from the total carbs in a food will give you its digestible or "net" carb content. For instance, if a cup of mixed vegetables contains 10 grams of carbs and 4 grams of fiber, its net carb count is 6 grams.

When people with diabetes consume too many carbs at a time, their blood sugar levels can rise to dangerously high levels.

Question: What is therapeutic nourishment treatment?

Answer: Medicinal nourishment treatment is an assistance given by a RD to make individual eating plans dependent on your needs and likes. For individuals with diabetes, restorative sustenance treatment has been appeared to improve diabetes the board. Medicare pays for therapeutic nourishment treatment for individuals with diabetes Outer connection On the off chance that you have protection other than Medicare, inquire as to whether it covers restorative sustenance treatment for diabetes.

Question: Will enhancements and nutrients help my diabetes?

Answer: No reasonable verification exists that taking dietary enhancements NIH outside connection, for example, nutrients, minerals, herbs, or flavors can help oversee diabetes.1 You may require supplements in the event that you can't get enough nutrients and minerals from nourishments. Chat with your human services supplier before you take any dietary enhancement since some can cause reactions or influence how your medications work.

Question: How might I be physically dynamic securely in the event that I have diabetes?

Answer: Physical action is a significant piece of dealing with your blood glucose level and remaining solid. Being dynamic has numerous medical advantages.

Physical action brings down blood glucose levels, circulatory strain, improves blood stream and burns out additional calories so you can hold your weight down if necessary. However, it improves your disposition and can forestall falls and improve memory in more seasoned grown-ups.

In the event that you are overweight, joining physical action with a decreased calorie eating plan can prompt significantly more advantages. In the Look Forward: Activity for Wellbeing in Diabetes study,1 overweight grown-ups with type 2 diabetes who ate less and moved more had more noteworthy long haul medical advantages contrasted with the individuals who didn't roll out these improvements. These advantages included improved cholesterol levels, less rest apnea, and having the option to move around more effectively.

Indeed, even limited quantities of physical movement can help. Specialists propose that you focus on at any rate 30 minutes of moderate or energetic physical action 5 days of the week.3 Moderate movement feels to some degree hard, and fiery action is extreme and feels hard. On the off chance that you need to get thinner or keep up weight reduction, you may need to complete an hour or a greater amount of physical movement 5 days of the week.

Show restraint. It might take half a month of physical action before you see changes in your wellbeing.

Make certain to drink water previously, during, and after exercise to remain all around hydrated. Coming up next are some different tips for safe physical movement when you have diabetes. Drink water when you exercise to remain very much hydrated.

Question: What physical activities should I do if I have diabetes?

Answer: Most kinds of physical activity can help you take care of your diabetes. Certain activities may be unsafe for some people, such as those with low vision or nerve damage to their feet. Ask your health care team what physical activities are safe for you. Many people choose walking with friends or family members for their activity.

Doing different types of physical activity each week will give you the most health benefits. Mixing it up also helps reduce boredom and lower your chance of getting hurt. Try these options for physical activity.

Question: When would it be advisable for me to eat in the event that I have diabetes?

Answer: A few people with diabetes need to eat at about a similar time every day. Others can be progressively adaptable with the planning of their dinners. Contingent upon your diabetes prescriptions or kind of insulin, you may need to eat a similar measure of starches simultaneously every day. In the event that you take "supper time" insulin, your eating timetable can be increasingly adaptable.

On the off chance that you utilize certain diabetes medications or insulin and you skip or postpone a supper, your blood glucose level can drop excessively low. Ask your medicinal services group when you ought to eat and whether you ought to eat when physical action.

Question: What amount would i be able to eat on the off chance that I have diabetes?

Answer: Eating the perfect measure of nourishment will likewise assist you with dealing with your blood glucose level and your weight. Your human services group can assist you with making sense of how a lot of nourishment and what number of calories you ought to eat every day.

Question: Going Low-Carb for Diabetes: Does It Work?

Answer: Carbs have been generally taken a gander at as the adversary of individuals with type 2 diabetes, yet they don't need to be. You can at present eat carbs — including grains — on a diabetes eating plan, says Palinkski-Swim. The key is to get those carbs from shrewd sources (entire grains, vegetables, natural product, dairy), limit your carb admission to close to 60 g for every supper (all in all), and space them out for the duration of the day for best glucose control.

However, in the event that you are keen on going low-carb, there is some proof that this kind of diet plan can be valuable to those with type 2 diabetes. For example, a fundamental research survey in 2017 found that a low-carb plan helped grown-ups with diabetes bring down their triglyceride levels and lift "great" HDL cholesterol. It might likewise have mind-body benefits, as individuals said they were less focused and more joyful between dinners. Another audit inferred that low-carb consumes less calories drop blood glucose levels and enable individuals to utilize less prescription, or dispose of it totally. The creators prescribe it as a first-line treatment for diabetes.

While the advantages are energizing, in the event that you do go low-carb, know about the dangers, which incorporate supplement lacks. You may likewise not get enough fiber in case you're not eating enough nonstarchy vegetables. Eating an excessive amount of protein can likewise bargain kidney wellbeing.

Question: What physical exercises would it be advisable for me to do in the event that I have diabetes?

Answer: Nourishment and physical action are significant pieces of a solid way of life when you have diabetes. Alongside different advantages, following a sound supper plan and being dynamic can assist you with keeping your blood glucose level, additionally called glucose, in your objective range. To deal with your blood glucose, you have to adjust what you eat and drink with physical movement and diabetes prescription, in the event that you take any. What you decide to eat, the amount you eat, and when you eat are immensely significant in keeping your blood glucose level in the range that your social insurance group suggests.

Getting progressively dynamic and causing changes in what you to eat and drink can appear to be trying from the outset. You may think that its simpler to begin with little changes and find support from your family, companions, and medicinal services group.

- Eating admirably and being physically dynamic most days of the week can support you
- Keep your blood glucose level, pulse, and cholesterol in your objective extents
- Get more fit or remain at a solid weight
- Forestall or defer diabetes issues
- Feel better and have more vitality

Question: What nourishments would i be able to eat on the off chance that I have diabetes?

Answer: You may stress that having diabetes implies abandoning nourishments you appreciate. Fortunately you can even now eat your preferred nourishments, yet you may need to eat littler segments or appreciate them less frequently. Your human services group will help make a diabetes dinner plan for you that addresses your issues and likes.

Question: Which nourishments ought to be kept away from in a type 2 diabetes Diet plan?

Answer: Individuals with type 2 diabetes ought to stay away from a large number of the equivalent undesirable nourishments everybody should restrain. Dietary limitations include: Soft drinks: both sugar improved standard pop and diet soft drink raise glucose.

Refined sugars (doughnuts, baked goods, cakes, treats, scones, desserts, sweet)

Question: What Are Some Eating routine Plans That May Profit Individuals With Type 2 Diabetes?

Answer: While it's ideal to converse with your primary care physician before beginning any eating regimen plan, it's particularly critical to converse with them in case you're keen on the accompanying:

Ketogenic Diet You'll eat not many carbs on this arrangement (20 to 50 g daily) to accomplish a condition of ketosis, where your body consumes fat for fuel rather than carbs. "There is some examination that recommends ketogenic diets may lessen insulin obstruction and improve blood glucose levels," says Palinski-Swim. Surely, one investigation of grown-ups with type 2 diabetes who followed a ketogenic diet for 10 weeks improved glycemic control and helped patients bring down their measurements of medicine. (26) Still, it's a disputable eating routine, so make a point to gauge the advantages and disadvantages with your doctor.

Discontinuous Fasting (IF) IF requests that you limit the time you eat to a specific number of hours of the day, or to eat a low number of calories on specific days. Also, restricted research (little investigations and creature preliminaries) have demonstrated advantages to fasting glucose and weight. So, skipping dinners may block glucose control or cause low glucose (hypoglycemia), particularly in case you're on insulin, so converse with your primary care physician about the dangers and advantages before endeavoring.

Paleo Diet The reason of this arrangement is to eat like our tracker gatherer precursors, concentrating on organic products, vegetables, nuts, lean meat, and certain fats. (It takes out grains, vegetables, and most dairy.) One investigation in 2015 found that both paleo eats less and the rules from the ADA improved glucose control in patients with type 2 diabetes — however the paleo weight watchers ended up as the winner.

Question: What Are the Best Well known Eating routine Designs for Individuals Overseeing Type 2 Diabetes?

Answer: Good dieting, following the rules beneath on building a diabetes dinner plan, and concentrating on settling on nutritious decisions more often than not can assist you with shedding weight. Working with an enrolled dietitian who is likewise a confirmed diabetes instructor can assist you with arriving at your objective weight while meeting the entirety of your wholesome needs.

So, you may like the course offered by an eating regimen plan. The two that are recommended for individuals with diabetes on numerous occasions are the Mediterranean eating regimen and the Scramble (Dietary Ways to deal with Stop Hypertension) diet. Not at all like purported "abstains from food" (a considerable lot of which are planned distinctly for the present moment), these eating approaches expect to set the establishment for building and keeping up deep rooted propensities.

Palinski-Swim supports the Mediterranean eating routine since "it's been examined for a considerable length of time and has been demonstrated to be advantageous at lessening the danger of coronary illness," she says. That is significant on the grounds that individuals with diabetes are up to multiple times bound to pass on from coronary illness contrasted and grown-ups without diabetes.

Following the Mediterranean eating regimen, you'll center around entire nourishments as products of the soil, entire grains, olive oil, vegetables, nuts, and poultry and fish, while constraining red meat.

Another eating regimen choice to consider is the Scramble diet. "The Scramble diet has been seen as gainful at lessening circulatory strain levels, a key hazard factor for coronary illness and kidney ailment. Since both of these ailment dangers are raised with diabetes, this style of eating may advance a decrease in the danger of comorbid conditions related with diabetes," Palinski-Swim clarifies.

Like the Mediterranean eating routine, the Scramble diet advances eating leafy foods, entire grains, fish and poultry, beans, nuts, just as without fat or low-fat dairy. You'll additionally top sodium to 2,300 milligrams (mg) every day (1,500 mg whenever prompted by a specialist).

Question: Why Is It Critical to Eat Well, When managing Diabetes, and What Are the Dangers on the off chance that You Don't?

Answer: Diabetes is described by a condition called insulin opposition, where the body can't successfully utilize the hormone insulin to ship (glucose) to cells and muscles for vitality. This makes glucose collect in your blood at higher than typical levels, which can place your wellbeing in harm's way.

Picking the perfect measures of the correct nourishments can assist lower with blooding sugar levels and keep them relentless, lessening diabetes manifestations and helping bring down the hazard for wellbeing complexities, for example, nerve harm, vision issues, coronary illness, kidney harm, and stroke.

Eating admirably can likewise assist you with losing and keep up a solid weight. Actually, losing only 5 to 7 percent of your body weight may assist you with bettering control type 2 diabetes, or forestall prediabetes from advancing into the all out type of the illness.

As opposed to attempting to update your way of life with handy solutions, make enduring propensities by concentrating on little, basic, and viable changes, Palinski-Swim says. Else, you may feel overpowered and return to your old, unfortunate eating ways — and recapture weight you've lost. "Being reliable with change, regardless of how little, is critical to long haul weight reduction achievement," she includes. Here are four to kick you off:

Pack in more veggies. Include one additional serving of nonstarchy vegetables at supper. Consider adding vegetables to a bite, as well.

Fit in more natural product. Research shows that eating berries, apples, and pears is related with weight reduction. Go figure, these are particularly fiber-rich decisions. Obviously, all different organic products tally, as well — simply make certain to consider them your starch servings.

Remain dynamic. Eventually, you should expect to be dynamic 150 minutes out of each week (that is only 30 minutes five days of the week). Be that as it may, at first, begin by strolling 15 minutes a couple of times each week, and including time from that point. This helpful diagram will tell you the best way to develop gradually.

Snack on something in the first part of the day. Having breakfast is one propensity for long haul weight-failures. A plain yogurt with organic product, nuts and natural product, or fried eggs and entire grain toast are all diabetes-accommodating morning meals.

Individuals who are overweight or large are at a more serious hazard for creating diabetes in any case. Being overweight or fat is likewise connected with expanded danger of conditions, for example, particular kinds of malignant growth, osteoarthritis, greasy liver malady, and the previously mentioned diabetes inconveniences.

Question: What nourishments and beverages would it be advisable for me to restrict in the event that I have diabetes?

Answer:

- Meals and beverages to confine incorporate
- Seared nourishments and different nourishments high in immersed fat and trans fat
- Meals high in salt, additionally called sodium
- Desserts, for example, heated products, treat, and frozen yogurt
- Refreshments with included sugars, for example, juice, normal pop, and customary games or caffeinated drinks
- Drink water rather than improved refreshments. Consider utilizing a sugar substitute in your espresso or tea.

On the off chance that you drink liquor, drink decently—close to one beverage daily in case you're a lady or two beverages per day in case you're a man. In the event that you use insulin or diabetes medications that expansion the measure of insulin your body makes, liquor can make your blood glucose level drop excessively low. This is particularly valid in the event that you haven't eaten in some time. It's ideal to eat some nourishment when you drink alcohol.